THINK THIN

30 Visualizations to Help You Lose Weight and Keep It Lost

by Valerie Wells

Chronicle Books ★ **San Francisco**

Printed in the United States of America

Library of Congress Cataloging-in-Publication Data
Wells, Valerie.
Think thin: 30 visualizations to help you lose weight and keep it lost
by Valerie Wells.
p.   cm.
ISBN: 0-8118-0089-X
1. Reducing. 2. Visualization. 3. Mind and body. I. Title.
RM222.2.W343 1992
613.2'5—dc20   91-34280
CIP
Cover & Book Design: Terry Irwin
Cover Illustration: Karen Smidth

Distributed in Canada by Raincoast Books
112 East Third Avenue, Vancouver, B.C. V5T 1C8

10 9 8 7 6 5 4 3 2 1

Chronicle Books
275 Fifth Street
San Francisco, CA 94103

Acknowledgments

Writing this book was like preparing a thirty-course dinner. I couldn't have done it without help in the writing kitchen from my friends who provided nourishing support and well-seasoned laughter.

I especially want to thank my literary agent, Heide Lange, for support above and beyond the call of duty. And my heartfelt gratitude to my spiritual mother, Leita Kaldi, for her caring and wisdom, and to my soul sister, Pat Weinman, for sharing Rivka. Many sweet thanks to:

Mark Clerkin	Mary Alice Mark
Harry Crews	Katerina Nadel
Rusty Erdman	Steve Narron
Gary Farmer	Scott Silverman
Richard Frankel	Howard Sloane
Irene Giersing	Cathy Steele
Kirby Hotchner	Terrence Tullgren
Jacques Lehrer	Linda Wilensky

Visualize me toasting you with a glass of sparkling cider, held high. May you each dine well and long at the feast of life.

And many thanks to the News Cafe, Rolos, and the Front Porch for allowing me space and time to write.

Contents

Part I

The Why And What of Visualization

How you look in your mind is how you'll look in the mirror. Think thin, and you'll be thin. See yourself as fat in your mind, and you'll see yourself as fat in the mirror. The mind-body connection makes it vitally important to lose the mental image of yourself as fat in order to lose physical pounds and keep them lost.

If you want to look thin, but continue to think that you're fat, you're headed for the yo-yo land of losing and gaining weight. An estimated 50 million Americans are overweight, with 20 million who are on diets at any one time. A large percentage of those who lose weight eventually regain some, all, or even more than the weight they lost. And then they diet again. And gain again. And diet again. And gain again. Some chronic dieters actually lose and gain their entire body weight several times over. One of the main reasons for this yo-yo phenomenon is that people shed pounds, but neglect to shed the old, limiting mental image of themselves as being overweight.

Your subconscious strives for consistency between physical and mental images, so when your image in the mirror looks thin, but the image in your mind looks fat, a conflict is created. Your subconscious is alerted and takes steps to correct the contradiction. It overrides the newer, more fragile physical image of being slim, in favor of the more vivid and deeply ingrained mental image of being overweight. Almost before you can say, "I am thin," your subconscious influences you to overeat. As Virgil said in the *Aeneid* almost two thousand years ago, "Mind moves matter." Your subconscious mind causes fat matter to move back onto your arms, waist, stomach, hips, buttocks, and thighs, resolving the conflict between thin and fat images.

Mind over matter works, and it means that your mind matters. The goal is to make your mind work *for* you instead of against you. By thinking thin, using the remarkably effective, yet fun and easy visualizations offered in this book, you can replace the image of yourself as overweight with a strong, vibrant image of yourself at your ideal weight. Once you achieve your ideal weight, visualization helps you maintain it.

The visualizations in *Think Thin* are designed to help you:

1. Create a strong, clear desire to lose weight.
2. Establish a positive and vivid mental image of yourself at your ideal weight.
3. Make losing weight easier and more enjoyable.
4. Help you gain control over your life and eating habits.
5. Enable you to cope successfully with fattening emotions.
6. Eliminate counterproductive beliefs and attitudes.
7. Help sustain weight loss.

Using visualization increases the effectiveness of diet and exercise programs. When you combine mental action with physical action, you create a synergy of success. By thinking thin you become thin more easily because you're reinforcing your diet, rather than being in conflict with it. Exercising your mind by visualizing how you want to look also increases the benefits you derive from exercising your body.

When you take effective action in your mental world, you increase your self-esteem as well as your ability to effect positive change in your physical world. The very act of visualizing brings a sense of calm, well-being, and confidence.

What is visualization? Basically it's a language that uses pictures instead of words. It could be called "picturese." This language of mental images is perceived with your mind's eye. But what if you think that your mindsight is less than 20/20? In all probability you're maintaining a belief that you can't visualize and it's clouding your mental vision. When you suspend the belief that you can't visualize, mental vision will improve.

Just about everyone has mental eyesight: try finding your keys, your car, or your way home without being able to see, or sense, a mental picture of what they look like and where they're located. By the age of seven months babies have been able to find a rattle hidden under a pillow, indicating that they had an image of the rattle in their minds that they matched with the physical image. Studies done by Jerome L. Singer of Yale University show that 96 percent of the population daydreams. The clarity with which you daydream is an indication of how well you see with your mind's eye.

If you can picture your front door, your best friend's face, or a pink elephant in a polka-dot skirt, be assured that you can visualize. Even if the image is fuzzy and out of focus, or long on outlines but short on details, as long as you have a recognizable sense of the image you can learn to communicate in "picturese."

"Picturese," or visualization, is the native language of your subconscious; words can be considered its second language. Your subconscious mind "speaks" in pictures and "hears" in pictures, so if you want to communicate effectively with it, visualization is the language of choice. Through the language of visualization your conscious mind and your subconscious mind can carry on a two-way conversation.

Why would you want to talk with your subconscious? Because it contains vital information about who you think you've been, who you think you are, and who you think you'll be. Your subconscious is like a vast and powerful computer that stores all the information your conscious mind puts into it in picture bytes. The stored experiences of your past and dreams for your future become programs that run, or define, your present.

Computer programmers have a saying: "Garbage in, garbage out." It means that if you put incorrect or out-moded information into a computer, that's what you'll get out. Ditto for your subconscious. If a past picture of yourself as fat is stored in the memory banks of your subconscious, then you'll be fat now and in the future. If you delete the limiting, outmoded images of yourself as fat, and replace them with bright mental pictures of yourself as thin, you'll be thin. You get out what you put in.

To help you understand the nature of your subconscious so you can achieve the slim and healthy body you desire, there are four other important characteristics that your subconscious shares with a computer.

1. Just like a computer, your subconscious is very literal. It will do what you tell it to, but you have to be very clear and specific; it isn't able to fill in the gaps, or second-guess you. Its response is based solely on the pictures and programs you have put into it. A computer cannot run a word processing program unless one has been loaded into its memory, and your subconscious can't run a thin program unless you've put one in. Until you create a "Thin" program, your subconscious will continue to act on the directives stored in your "Fat" program.

2. Both your subconscious and a computer have certain directives that determine how they function. One of the primary directives of your subconscious is consistency: images of the same thing must match. If the physical image and the mental image don't match, an error message flashes. In order to maintain consistency the weaker image changes to match the stronger image. If you're fat but create a strong, steady mental image of being thin, your physical reality will change to match your mental reality.

3. In a computer, all information exists in the present, even when notated with a past or future date, and it doesn't fade over time. The same is true of your subconscious. In your subconscious, every image and every

piece of data that is stored exists in the present. Although your conscious mind dates an image as being in the past or in the future, that image exists in your subconscious in the here and now with all its original clarity. That's why you can think of a sad experience from the past and feel sad now, or feel happy thinking about an enjoyable future event. When you give your subconscious a clear picture of you being thin, it registers in your subconscious as the present, and your eating behavior aligns with the thin image.

4. Whether you feed a computer a photograph of a tree or use the computer and your imagination to create a picture of a tree, both pictures appear equally real to the computer. In the same way, images from your physical world and images from your imagination appear equally real to your subconscious. Your subconscious scans primarily for form, content, and intensity, and can't tell the difference between physical and mental realities. Did you ever think about biting into a fresh lemon and salivate? Or recall the sound of nails on a blackboard and feel a shiver in your spine? Or wake from a vivid dream, momentarily unsure of where you are and what has "really" taken place? You react as if the thought were a physical reality. When you create a convincing mental image of being thin, your subconscious will register it as reality and support thin behavior.

Together, these four key characteristics can help unlock the power of your mind. When it comes to making changes, they are essential to making your subconscious your ally, not your enemy. If you want your body to weigh less, but you've only stored images of yourself weighing more, your subconscious will continue to influence your behavior based on the images of being overweight. To lose weight successfully it is necessary to consciously delete the "Think Fat" program that's been running your behavior, and consciously load a program into your subconscious entitled "Think Thin."

This can be accomplished through the visualizations in this book. As soon as you begin to think thin, you'll begin to become thin because your mental state directly affects your physical state. You are what you think you are. The effect of the mind on the body is dramatically evident in the fields of sports and health.

A recorded observation of the mind affecting the body was made in the 1920s by American physiologist Edmund Jacobson. First he measured the electrical activity of his subjects when their bodies were at rest. Then he told them to visualize themselves running. When Jacobson measured the electrical activity of his subjects while they were visualizing, he discovered that the muscles associated with running contracted in small, but detectable, amounts.

In his book, *Psycho-Cybernetics*, published in 1960, Maxwell Maltz tells of golf instructor Alex Morrison, who developed a system of golf practice that took place entirely in a golfer's mind. Without ever walking out on a green, or wrapping a hand around a club, golfers were able to improve their handicap just by sitting in an armchair and visualizing themselves adapting an ideal stance and swinging smoothly to make the ball arc down the fairway.

Visualizing successful athletic performance primarily affects the voluntary muscles, but visualization has also been shown to affect the autonomic nervous system that controls the involuntary muscles. During a laboratory study, a yogi named Swami Rama was able to create different temperatures on two sides of his palm by mentally willing it. He was also able to stop his heart for twenty seconds, then start it again.

In medicine, the powerful connection between body and mind was recognized long ago by the Egyptians, and was respected until the seventeenth century, when the advances of industry and technology made machines appear to be more efficient and effective than the mind. Recently, however, doctors have come to realize that worry and stress can adversely affect the body, causing ulcers, high blood pressure, and heart conditions. Many patients who have used mental relaxation methods and biofeedback have been able to reduce high blood pressure, control migraine headaches, and ease muscle tension.

Carl and Stephanie Simonton took the effect of the mind on the body a step farther, using visualization as a powerful tool to help terminally ill cancer patients at their Cancer Counseling and Research Center in Fort Worth, Texas. Patients successfully used mental imagery to mobilize and strengthen their immune systems and rout out cancer cells. Although doctors had given up all hope for their recovery, many patients' cancer went into remission.

Such health and athletic improvements are possible because the subconscious mind doesn't distinguish between mental reality and physical reality, or between the past and the future; it's your conscious mind that makes those distinctions. When you create a mental image of the future that's vivid and charged with emotion, your subconscious responds to it as if it were physically real and happening in the present.

Evidence is mounting that you can direct your thoughts to have positive impact on the health and performance of your body. This makes visualization a powerful tool in helping you create mental images for losing weight. Think thin and be thin!

Part II

How, When, and Where to Visualize

The thirty visualizations in *Think Thin* represent a month's supply of healthy, nutritious, nonfattening images to feed your mind. Think of them as food for thought. Visualizing yourself thin is an effective, yet fun way to change your mind about your body, and thus change your body. Used in conjunction with diet and exercise, thinking thin enhances their benefits. Each visualization offers insight and provides a creative course of action for change.

Designed to be entertaining in order to grab the attention of both your conscious and subconscious minds, the visualizations imprint positive weight-loss images on both levels. Your subconscious, in particular, is more apt to notice images that are vivid, fun, and emotionally bright. If you think of your mind as a picture gallery of information, you can imagine how the attention of your subconscious would be drawn more to a lovingly photographed, colorful image charged with positive emotion than to a drab black and white photo of something indeterminate.

Another image quality that engages the attention of your subconscious is that of something unusual or unexpected taking place in a familiar context. For instance, the image of a swimming pool is familiar, but to have it full of money with a happy bear swimming in it makes your subconscious sit up and take notice. If the pool tiles are engraved with your initials and the bear is wearing polka dots, even better.

Once the image you create in your conscious mind has the attention of your subconscious, you can have a two-way conversation. The visualizations in *Think Thin* enable you to speak "picturese," the native language of your subconscious, so you can both talk to your subconscious and hear what it says. Each visualization supplies the gist of what to say and how to say it, and also provides your subconscious with a format for responding.

You speak picturese by consciously projecting an image, and your subconscious replies by making either positive or negative changes in the image. This feedback is extremely valuable because it lets you know whether the images stored in the memory banks of your subconscious will help or hinder you in achieving your goal.

For instance, when you picture the pool with the bear swimming in money, if hindering beliefs that you don't deserve to have money are stored in your memory banks, your subconscious might reply with a picture of a sad brown bear standing forlornly at the bottom of an empty pool. Receiving this image doesn't mean that you're a bad person and doomed to poverty, it's just your subconscious alerting you to the fact that the way you see yourself with regard to money is limiting.

Being aware that a limiting image is stored is invaluable, because the first step in resolving a problem is knowing that it exists. When you receive an image that contradicts the one you sent, use visualization to tell your subconscious to erase the limiting image and replace it with an image of success.

Talking to your subconscious is the same as talking to someone you want to get an important point across to: you speak distinctly, in an interesting way, and use words they understand. In the case of talking to your subconscious, the more you can articulate the image, and the more fun and colorful the details, the better your subconscious will understand you. You'll know that your subconscious has gotten the picture when its response to your picture of the pool and the bear is a picture of the pool overflowing with money and the bear is doing the backstroke.

The same conversational process holds true when visualizing yourself as thin. You might tell your subconscious that you want to be thin by means of a picture of you standing on a scale showing your ideal weight. Your subconscious might reply with an image of the scale showing you weighing the same, or even more. This doesn't mean that you're a bad person doomed to fatness, it's just your subconscious mind telling your conscious mind that stored images of yourself as fat will hinder you from becoming thin.

Change your image. Use visualization to clearly and emphatically tell your subconscious that the old limiting image is to be replaced with a new image of you weighing X number of pounds. When your subconscious replies with an image of you standing on a scale at the top of a mountain with a rainbow arcing overhead, and the number

19

of pounds you want to weigh is flashing in neon colors, then you know that the new image has been heard.

Visualization allows your conscious mind and your subconscious mind to have an informative and creative conversation. You make visual statements and ask questions, and your subconscious replies. There are no wrong answers. Whatever picture your subconscious responds with is the truth as the subconscious sees it. It's important to remember that your subconscious is literal, like a computer, and not sarcastic or mean, so the images with which it replies are neither judgments nor criticisms, but simply information that's been stored in its memory banks.

The tone of these visualizations is often childlike because your subconscious is most receptive to information that is simply told. Some visualizations are short, with a single, simple theme. Others are longer and more intricate, providing several levels to explore and several options to choose from. You can also mix and match the images. You might want to combine "Scaling Down" with "Thinabration," or "Fat Elves" with "Restaurant of Your Dreams."

The beauty of using visualizations to explore and change your inner world is that the images never become stale or used up. As you change and evolve, so do the images. For instance, your Palace of Power will appear one way initially, and then as your confidence and imagination increase, its appearance and resources will likewise change and grow.

Make these visualizations your own. Adapt and adopt them to your particular needs and creative inclinations. A visualization is just a blueprint for the mind, but once constructed you can furnish and decorate it the way you want, even changing its size and shape. Make each visualization pleasant to be in by including details that make you happy. Avoid making the visualizations difficult, or you'll give your subconscious the message that losing weight is difficult. Make the visualizations work by playing with them. When the images are fun and easy, losing weight will be fun and easy.

There are several ways to choose a visualization from among the thirty offered. Because this is a one-month's supply of visualizations, you can do one a day like a vitamin, beginning with number 1, "Seed of Desire," and ending with number 30, "Thinabration." Or look at the Contents and simply pick a title that appeals to you. Or leaf through the pages, reading visualizations until you find one that tickles your fancy. If you want to be spontaneous, open the book at random and read the visualization the pages open to.

Once you've chosen a visualization, read it over a couple of times in order to become familiar with the concept and the sequence of images so you can do it on your own. (Because you'll be reading the visualizations instead of listening to someone guide you through, don't expect to be lulled into a relaxed alpha state.) The advantage to doing the visualizations consciously, and being your own guide, is that you can take as little or as much time with various segments as you want. If a particular aspect of a visualization intrigues you, you can explore it to your heart's and mind's content.

When you're able to remember the flow of images in a *Think Thin* visualization you can do it anywhere, anytime you have a couple of minutes:

- upon waking, while still in bed
- bathing
- on an exercise bike
- during meals
- between meals
- stopped at a red light
- on a bus
- during work breaks
- on hold on the telephone
- waiting for an appointment
- working out
- jogging
- bicycling
- waiting in line
- in bed, before going to sleep

As you become familiar with several visualizations, you'll have a colorful assortment in mind to choose from, wherever you are.

When visualizing, your eyes can be open or closed, depending on where you are and what you're doing. Many people prefer visualizing with their eyes closed because they find they can concentrate better on their mental environment if they're not distracted by the sight of their physical environment. Some people have reported that visualizing while on an exercise bike not only makes the time fly by, but also seems to energize the images.

The more often you reinforce a positive image, the more clearly it is heard by your subconscious, and the more vividly it is imprinted in its memory banks. The more the information stored in your subconscious agrees with your conscious goals, the more you'll get what you want. Think thin happily and often, and you'll be thin.

For best results, avoid making the visualization process arduous and tedious. The quality and spirit of your effort is what's most important. It's more effective to enliven the image with clear desire and bright imagination for three to five minutes than to drag it out half-heartedly for an hour. Have you ever waited for someone to take your picture, and they ditzed around for so long adjusting the camera that your enthusiasm waned and your smile froze? That's the effect that prolonging the visualization beyond the moment of bright enthusiasm can have on your subconscious.

Try taking three quick, colorful pictures a day with the camera of your mind. Visualize the image you've chosen for just a couple of minutes when you first wake up, to start your day with a positive focus. Then visualize again during the middle of the day to reinforce the image, and once more at night just before you fall asleep, as a final reminder to your subconscious.

Use a visualization for whatever length of time you want. You might like the variety of doing two or three a day. Or you might want to use a particular visualization as a focus for the whole day, or even for a week. You'll know what works best by the images your subconscious replies with, and, of course, by the quantity and quality of what you're eating.

These visualizations are effective, yet fun, so have a good time with them. The more fun you have, the better the results, because when your subconscious is having a good time it's more eager to help you achieve your goal of being thin.

The more often you think thin,
The more vividly your thin image is imprinted on
your subconscious,
And the more easily you'll be thin!

Learning how to visualize is one instance in which something is actually easier done than said. You don't need any special equipment to visualize, just three basic tools:

1. A mind.
2. A heart.
3. A will (as in "where there's a will, there's a way").

If you're able to add two plus two, feel glad to see a friend, and get yourself up in the morning, you already possess all three. Equipped with these three tools, you're ready to visualize.

The mechanics of visualization are similar to those of a camera. Your mind is like the lens of a camera that frames and focuses the desired image. Your positive emotions are the flash of light that illuminates the image. And your subconscious is the film on which the image is imprinted. Here are four basic steps to taking a good visualization picture.

Four Steps of Visualization

1. *SEE THE GOAL.* It's as important to aim your mental camera at the goal you want as it is to aim a real camera at whatever it is you want to take a picture of. Say you want a picture of sweet Aunt Millie standing in front of her house, but you're lackadaisical about where you aim the camera; you could wind up with a spiffy photo of her elbow, the lawn, the house next door, or the sky. Those might not be bad pictures, but they're not the picture you wanted.

The goal you want to take a picture of is you being happily thin. Make sure you have a clear shot. If someone is standing in your way, tell him or her to move. If anything is blocking your shot, remove it.

Form as clear a mental picture as possible in order for a sharp image to be imprinted on the film of your subconscious. Use your mind's eye to bring the images in each visualization into sharp focus. If you can't see it, sense it. Compose details. Highlight colors. Extend the depth of field. It's also important to see yourself clearly in each visualization so your subconscious knows that this goal's for you.

You'll find that you can focus your mental pictures more clearly if you're relaxed. Being tense when you visualize causes the camera of your mind to shake, which blurs the image. So, before visualizing, r-e-e-l-a-a-a-x. Try stamping your feet a couple of times to ground yourself, then shake out tension through your hands. Take a slow, deep breath. Get mentally loose.

2. *FEEL THE GOAL.* You used your mind to *see* yourself in the picture, now use your heart to *feel* yourself in the picture. Participate with all your senses. You have the mental equivalent of all your physical senses, so use them to get right inside the image. See, hear, smell, taste, and touch the image to make it come alive, experiencing it as if it were actually happening. Feel the excitement of having what you want. Feel the pleasure and satisfaction that success brings. Positive emotions illuminate the goal.

Keeping your mind from wandering is just as important when experiencing the image as it is when focusing on it. If you start thinking about someone you're angry with, or thinking that you're going to fail, you'll wind up with the equivalent of a spiffy photo of a passing garbage truck instead of a happily thin you. Such negative emotions will darken your positive picture, and can even overshadow it completely, so keep both your mind and your heart focused on your goal. The fuller and richer your emotional experience, the better the visualization works.

3. *PRESS THE SHUTTER BUTTON.* Once you've framed and focused your goal with your mind and put your heart into it, you're ready to press the shutter button using the finger of desire. Allow your heartfelt desire for what you've pictured to build and intensify. Desire it openly and strongly. Then, in a flash of loving desire, snap the picture. *Click. Snap. Pop.* The shutter between your conscious mind and your subconscious mind opens, and the

flash of positive emotion illuminates the image, imprinting it on the film of your subconscious.

As soon as you feel the mental and emotional intensity peak, take your mental eye off the image. Go blank, or focus on something else, so that only the sharpest and brightest image is imprinted on your subconscious. Don't overexpose the image, or blur it with a double exposure.

4. *GET THE PICTURE.* Aligning your mind and heart with a goal increases your willingness to succeed. Increase it even more by giving yourself permission for the visualization to work. Consciously allowing success to happen is like developing the film.

If you don't believe that the visualization will work, or have a negative attitude about it, the picture won't develop properly, if at all. Having doubts and fears is like pouring acid on film.

Believe that the visualization will work with as much conviction as you believe that the sun will come up in the morning. And believe that you deserve to have it succeed as much as you deserve to breathe. Trust in your ability to visualize, and in the power of visualization.

When you use your mind to form a mental picture of your goal and your heart to experience it, you create a synergy of success. You're ready to pick up your photo.

Get the picture?

Four Steps to Successful Visualization

1. See your goal
2. Feel your goal
3. Press the shutter button
4. Get the picture

Visualizations

Fortis Imaginatio Generat Causum
"A strong imagination begets the event itself."

Seed of Desire

Desire initiates change. It defines the changes sought and puts them into motion. Desire itself is born of want or need:

> *I want to change my T-shirt because I prefer to wear a different color.*
> *I need to change my T-shirt because it's dirty.*

> •

> *I want to change jobs because I think I can realize more of my potential and achieve greater satisfaction in a different work structure.*
> *I need to change jobs because I need to earn more money.*

> •

> *I want to lose weight because I'll enjoy looking more attractive and feeling healthier.*
> *I need to lose weight because it's damaging my health.*

Whether you want to lose weight, or need to lose it, the desire to weigh less than you do now is the basis for all the changes you seek. Desire is at the heart of change; it is the seed from which change grows.

Using your mind's eye and your heart's hand, see and feel your seed of desire to lose weight. Where is it? In your mind? In your heart? In your stomach? In the palm of your hand? In your littlest toe on your right foot? Or is it somewhere outside you?

Wherever it is, find it. It might be as small as a caraway seed, or as big as a coconut. The size doesn't matter because every seed contains all the nutrients and power it needs to grow. What color is the seed? Black? Brown? Green? White? Pink? Turquoise? Gold?

What shape is the seed? Round? Oblong? Flat? Bean-shaped? Star-shaped? Heart-shaped? Or like an S for slim?

Touch the seed of your desire with your heart's hand. Is it warm or cool? Smooth or fuzzy? Soft or hard? Feel it vibrate with stored energy. Feel the love for life the seed holds. This seed of desire to lose weight represents a part of you that loves you and wants you to be happy and healthy.

Wherever you find your seed of desire, ask it if that's where it wants to be planted. You'll have a feeling, or hear a word with your mind's ear, that will let you know if the seed wants to stay where it is, or be moved to a more fertile spot. If you found the seed of desire outside you, you will probably want to plant it within you. In your heart's hand, tenderly carry the seed to the place where it wants to be planted.

What does the place of planting look like? Is it a garden of wondrously colored, fragrant flowers? A field of fertile loam where rows of vegetables grow in healthy profusion? A special spot in a meadow? The banks of a sparkling river? A mountaintop? An ocean bed where sea anemones wave and cosmically colored parrot fish cruise by? Will you plant your seed in a crystal wand, a ball of shimmering light, or on an inner world in a galaxy known only to you?

Caringly plant your seed of desire in its chosen spot. You may bury it well beneath the surface, or gently push it in just a little way.

Water your seed of desire with gratitude. Be thankful that it exists, for without it the change you seek would not be possible. Be glad that there is a part of you that cares about your well-being.

Shine the warm bright light of joy on the seed of your desire to lose weight: joy for the vitality it contains. Joy for the future; the gift of a better life your desire brings you.

As you water your seed of desire with gratitude, and shine the light of joy upon it, the seed sprouts, its tip poking through the ground. Feel it putting down deep, strong roots within you, so that your desire to lose weight cannot easily be dislodged. Stems lengthen and leaves unfurl, until your desire is a sturdy tree growing within you, its trunk aligned with your spine, its limbs within your limbs. Does your desire blossom with fragrant flowers, or does it bear luscious fruit? As desire grows, it carries the oxygen needed to lose weight to every part of your body, and absorbs the carbon monoxide of wasteful thoughts and emotions.

Every area within you feels refreshed and strengthened with resolve to lose weight. See your desire grow in your heart, your mind, your stomach, the palm of your hand, down to the littlest toe of your right foot.

Keep your desire to lose weight alive and strong with daily care. Doubt, fear, anger, and resentment are like acid rain to desire. If you feel your desire weakening, visualize the place where you planted your seed of desire. Your subconscious will tell you the condition of your desire by showing you a mental picture of how it looks. If the blossoms are closed and drooping, or the fruit is beginning to rot, or the leaves are turning brown, prune as needed. Then water with gratitude and let the light of joy shine so that your desire to lose weight continues to be strong and healthy.

Skinny Dipping

Isn't it amazing how pants that come back from the laundry seem to have shrunk? That ol' zipper just doesn't slide up—you have to pull and tug. In case you have a sneaking suspicion that it might be you and not the pants, here's a way to see a slimmer you—and so *be* a slimmer you.

Imagine that you're standing on the bank of your own private stream. Scattered along the banks, and peeking out from the roots of trees, are bright spring flowers: daffodils, tulips, and lilies-of-the-valley. Robins and sparrows sing in the trees. Butterflies flutter and float nearby. A soft breeze stirs through your hair. The warmth of the sun sits comfortingly on your shoulders. Take off your shoes and wiggle your bare feet in the earth; blades of grass tickle your toes.

Before you the stream shimmers in the sunlight, flowing gently from right to left. Unable to resist the invitation of the pure, gleaming water, you decide to take a dip in the stream. You look around to make sure that you're alone, and take off your clothes. At first you feel a little self-conscious, but as you undress, a feeling of daring grabs you and you fling your clothes, letting them fall where they may.

Naked, you plunge into the stream. The water feels refreshingly clean and comfortable. The stream is no wider than you can easily swim, and no deeper than you are tall, so you feel safe being in the water. You float, and play, and splash in the stream. The more you enjoy the water, the happier you become. You feel mighty good about taking the plunge.

As you frolic in the water, you become aware that your body feels noticeably lighter. With pleasant surprise you realize that the water is softening your fat cells, and pounds of fat are literally melting away from every area of your body that you wish were thinner. What does the fat look like? What color is it? What consistency? As the fat melts off it's swept away by the current. You feel buoyant and carefree. The more you cavort happily in the water, the lighter you become.

As you're being cleaned by the stream, you glance at the bank on which your old clothes are strewn, and then look across to the opposite bank. From a tree branch hangs a brand-new outfit on a hanger. A tag is spindled over the hook of the hanger and flutters in the breeze. On it is written, in large block letters, your last name and first initial.

Curious, you swim easily across the stream to the opposite bank. Refreshed and slimmer, you climb up on the opposite bank. You move more fluidly and feel lighter on your feet. Then something wonderful and unique happens. You *see* the new you as if you were still standing in the stream. Seen from behind, your naked silhouette is definitely narrower. Your waist nips in, your buttocks are higher, and your thighs are more streamlined. You notice how differently you move. Take a moment to appreciate the improvements you see.

Then return your focus to how wonderful it feels being inside your thinner body. Merge completely with your lighter and tighter self. Jump up and down and skip around. Your new thinner body feels delightfully carefree and comfortable. Think about how much you're going to enjoy life. Thank the stream for carrying away those pounds, and give yourself a pat on your (now thinner) back for taking the plunge.

Look at your new clothes. They're exactly the style and color that are most flattering for you. As you take them off the hanger you notice that they're a size smaller than the clothes you left strewn about on the other bank. Slip them on. Everything fastens and zips with ease around the new slimmer you. Kick up your heels and do a happy little "skinny-dip" jig on the bank of your skinny stream.

Whenever you want to lose weight, the stream is there waiting to melt those pounds away. Just visualize the sparkling water and go skinny-dipping.

Palace of Power

You are the reigning monarch of your life, overseeing all that goes on in your kingdom. In order to solve problems, salve wounds (physical and otherwise), take constructive action, and make progress, an inner kingdom of calm and security is essential.

Reigning over your life is a full-time job, and you need a place of power where you can retreat in safety and comfort to focus your mind, explore its possibilities, garner information, and energize yourself. This visualization will help you create a specific place of power in your mindscape where you can make your dreams come true. You can travel there simply by picturing it.

What does your inner refuge look like? Some might think that a lean-to would do, and it might indeed be calm, but will it provide safety and room for exploration? Not likely. You're the king or queen of your life—isn't a full-fledged palace appropriate? Such a palace would protect, comfort, and allow room for growth in the manner to which you would like to become accustomed. You deserve it!

Take your first look at your palace from a vantage point about half a mile away. You're sitting astride a magnificent steed on a promontory overlooking your domain.

Your eyes scan the verdant lawns and gardens surrounding your palace. Forests teem with wildlife and healing herbs. A lake is abundant with fish, maybe even a couple of dolphins.

Nestled gracefully in the center is your palace. What design is it? It might be English, French, Italian, Austrian, Russian, or Moroccan, with two or more stories. It could be a combination palace and Disney castle. It could be a futuristic globe shape, all white, or be made of gold, or silver, or copper.

Seeing your palace makes you long to be there. You've been out surveying your kingdom and solving problems and could use some rest and relaxation. You press your heels into the horse's sides, and he takes off—literally. From the edge of the bluff he takes a powerful leap into the air, tail and mane streaking straight out, then lands gracefully at a full gallop, hardly jarring you at all. Feel the horse's power beneath you as his hooves fly swiftly and surely across the ground, carrying you home.

Arriving at your Palace of Power you find that, like a castle, it has a protective moat. The moat not only keeps out unwanted people, it also prevents negative events and thoughts from entering. Two guards stationed by the entry door lower the drawbridge, and you ride across, the sounds of your horse's hooves echoing against the water and the walls of the palace. At the door you dismount, giving your horse to a stable groom to feed and water.

Looking up, you see two silk banners hanging from poles over the large entry door. One has your name on it and a symbol of good fortune: a star, a horseshoe, a rainbow, or your own favorite good-luck symbol. The other banner proclaims PALACE OF POWER. With a wave to the guards you pass through the heavy double doors, noticing how reassuringly thick the walls of the palace are. What with the moat, the guards, and the thick walls, no one is going to get inside your palace unless they're invited.

The heavy doors close behind you and you find yourself in a high-ceilinged vestibule. How is it decorated? Of what material is the floor made? Does the light come from windows or from torches? Leave something of yours on a chair in the vestibule, or in a bowl on the table: a hat, a scarf, a ring, a notebook. You'll pick it up when you leave the palace.

Hanging from poles in the walls overhead are more silken banners. They bear such words as *Living Room, Dining Room, Kitchen, Library, Dream Chamber, Energy Arcade, Health Spa, Courtyard of Love, Money Pool, Valuarium, Basement of Beliefs,* and *Power Central,* each with an arrow pointing left, right, up, or down. You can go to any of these magical rooms and areas and avail yourself of their resources whenever you want.

To show you around and help you, a guide has been assigned to you. He or she enters from a side door, walks over to you, and stands by your side. What does he or she look like? How young or old? How short or tall? Your palace guide might look like Yoda or Alice in Wonderland. Or Merlin, or Wonder Woman. On the front of his or her clothes is embroidered the word Pal. On the back is embroidered a large ace of hearts.

Your palace guide is a most special Pal who will help you ace any situation. He or she will keep pace with you wherever you go, making sure you don't lose your way, and provide you with helpful hints whenever you need them. What a pal! Greet your Pal warmly, and thank him or her for being there for you.

The first thing your Pal does is remove your outerwear. If you're wearing armor it's removed and shined. If you're dusty and feeling less than fair, you're dusted off and shined. Your Pal places a soft warm cape about your shoulders. What color is the cape? Does it have a hood? As you lace the ties around your neck, your Pal tells you that this is your cape of power. It will protect you against the elements (physical and otherwise), warming you when it's cold, and keeping you cool when it's too hot.

From an array of thinking caps designed for various purposes, your Pal places a thinking cap on your head to help focus your thoughts. What does it look like? Thank your Pal for the cape and the cap.

Where do you want to go in the palace? The Dream Chamber banner has an arrow pointing up to the top floor. You decide to save that for later, but you do feel a trifle tired, so you head for the Energy Arcade. Following an arrow that points straight ahead, you come to a hall illuminated by seven round skylights, each with different-colored glass.

The first skylight is red casting a red circle, on the floor. Your Pal suggests that you stand in the center of the red circle for ten seconds. Standing on the circle, you're bathed in the red glow from the skylight. The color red seems to seep in through your skin, filling you with vitality. Walk to the next circle, which is orange, and bathe in the orange light, absorbing its creative energy into your body. The next circle is yellow, and the yellow light refreshes your mind. The green light fills you with love, and the blue makes you feel expressive. The lavender light revitalizes your spirit. At the end of the hall is a skylight of clear glass, and beneath it is a throne on which to sit, so that you can be filled and surrounded by bright white light.

What style is your throne? It might be white brocade or plush red velvet. It might be solid gold, silver filigree, smooth marble, or beautifully carved and polished wood. It could be made of a space-age alloy in an abstract shape. See and sense it in as much detail as possible.

There's a throne in every room of your palace. It might be the same style throne, or there might be a different style to suit each different room. This is your seat of power, so sit your seat down in it. Feel how comfortable your throne is. It supports and protects you. It energizes and inspires you. Wherever you are, your seat of power is.

The Energy Arcade and the power of your throne have helped to energize you. You feel renewed after your long journey and, with a flourish, you swirl your cape around you, doffing your cap to your Pal. Then, because pangs of hunger are gnawing at your stomach, you ask your Palace Pal to please show you to the Dining Room. There a table awaits you, laden with a smorgasbord of fresh fruits from your orchard, fresh vegetables from your gardens, and whatever other fresh foods appeal to you. The breads and cakes are from your bakery. Help yourself to whatever food you want, including dessert.

Your throne has been pulled up to a table covered with a lace cloth embroidered with the initials P.O.P., for Palace of Power, intertwined with your initials. Vases of fresh flowers from your gardens adorn the table. Waiters and waitresses wait nearby to bring you anything you want. Are they people, animals, or cartoon characters? Of what design are their uniforms?

A place has been set for you with goldware and crystal. Before sitting down you ask that a place be set for your Pal. A waiter or waitress pops out with a place setting and a napkin embroidered with P.A.L. and an ace of hearts. When you sit down to eat, your napkin is placed in your lap, along with a bag of gold coins.

Thirsty, you ask for something to drink. Out pops a waiter with a frosted glass of sparkling cider the color of pale ale lit with sunshine. You drink a toast to your Palace of Power, your Palace Pal, and to life. The cider leaps down your throat and bubbles into your body, filling every cell with sweet light.

You eat a little of this and a little of that, in any order you choose, pacing yourself so you don't overeat. The hearty flavors satisfy your taste buds, and the freshness of the food enlivens you. But before you feel full, you push your plate away. You feel completely nourished, infused with a sense of peace and well-being. The waiters and waitresses clap, applauding your mastery in the Dining Room. The palace bells peal.

From the Dining Room windows you look out on a heart-shaped Courtyard of Love. At the apex of the heart is a waterfall of diamonds splashing into a pool of serenity. Monarch butterflies flutter by fragrant flowers, gliding on orange and black wings. Where is your throne, and what style is it? The heart of your palace is so lovely to behold that it lovifies your own heart.

Energized and nourished, you can go anywhere in your palace and do anything with anyone. For instance, you may want to enjoy the Courtyard of Love privately, or you may want to invite someone you love to share its pleasures.

The same is true for your Money Pool, which is so large that there's a bear swimming in it, doing the backstroke. Frolic in your money pool, just you and the bear, or invite your family and friends for an enriching swim.

When you want knowledge, go to the Library. Everything you want to know is available to you there on books, computers, projectors, tapes, cassettes, slides, and so on. If you don't know where to look, ask your Pal for help.

Go to the Basement of Beliefs, where there's an alphabetized ledger of your beliefs about every aspect of your life, including your weight. Tear out the negative beliefs and replace them with handwritten positive beliefs.

The Valuarium is a sun-filled area on the roof, where you go to acknowledge the qualities about yourself that are of value to you and to others. This isn't the ego conceit of being better than others, it's simply recognizing your merits in order to nourish your self-esteem.

In the landscape of your mind and heart you have now established a place for your Palace of Power. Go there to prepare your mind for whatever you want to do in life. In your Palace of Power you can focus your mind and your energy to achieve weight loss and other goals as well. What your mind can conceive, you can receive.

To go to your Palace of Power, all you need to do is visualize yourself at the palace door, and you're there. As soon as your subconscious sees the image of the Palace of Power, it goes on alert, ready to give you whatever information you require. Certain elements and activities in the Palace attract the attention of your subconscious, and are therefore especially powerful. *Place* is important. Your *pal* is an *ace* of a friend. Having a *cape* and a *cap* is most helpful. To *leap* and yet *pace* yourself is good, as is to *clap* and hear bells *peal*. To quench your thirst, *pale ale* set on *lace* hits the spot. Having a *lap* in which to receive what you ask for is essential. Do it all, and use it all, and all will fall into your you-know-what.

With your Pal, explore the various rooms of power, creating new ones as the need arises. The more time you spend in your palace, the more powerful it becomes. Add power to other visualizations by first going to your Palace of Power and selecting a room or area that is appropriate for doing that particular visualization. In your Palace of Power you are the monarch, reigning over both your inner and outer kingdoms.

Lovified

Sometimes we eat not because we're hungry for food, but because we're hungry for love. Maybe we've come to believe that we're unlovable, and the belief continues to separate us from love, causing us to starve. Food is often the handiest substitute for love, and we stuff our faces when it is really our empty hearts that need filling. The next time your hunger pangs are in your heart, not in your stomach, fill up on this visualization instead of food.

Begin by picturing a brightly glowing ball of light somewhere in front of you. This is the universal light of love, which inspires growth and illuminates. You might see the light as bright white, or pink, or a rainbow swirl of all the colors of love.

How far away from you is love? It might be close, or it might be only a dot on the horizon. A road stretches from you to love. What is the condition of the road to love? Allow the image of it to surface honestly. Is it smooth going or do boulders block the way? Are there brambles that scratch and tear? Will potholes cause you to go flat, or send you careening out of control? Will you run into a brick wall? Are there nails to puncture you, or road blocks to impede you? Is there a toll booth at which you must pay a price for love?

What season is it in love country? Spring? Summer? Autumn? Winter? What's the weather like? Clear skies and sunshine? Cloudy skies and rain? Thunder and lightening? Fog? Snow? Hail?

The conditions you see between you and love reflect how you see yourself in regard to love. If the road is hilly and twisty and there are several obstacles, you either see yourself as being difficult to love, or believe that love is difficult. Barriers can also be defenses against being hurt by love, just as an overabundance of fat can deter love and insulate you against the pain of love.

Take a chance on love. Maybe this lovelight won't hurt. Maybe it will even fill you up. Clear the way between you and love.

Straighten, smooth, and level the road. Blast the boulders into gravel. Burn the brambles to ashes. Fill the potholes. Put an opening in the brick wall, or demolish it entirely. Remove nails with a large magnet. Push over barricades. Close the toll booth, putting up a sign that says FREE LOVE, so that love is both free and at liberty.

Let there be clear skies and sunshine. Feel a gentle breeze against your cheek. See flowers and fruit trees gracing the landscape.

Love is in sight, and you've cleared the way to it. Now decrease the distance between you and love by moving toward it. How do you move? Do you take hesitant baby steps? Do you walk with purpose? Do you skip with glee? Do you run with enthusiasm? Do you glide with grace? Do you float with joy?

As you move toward love, love moves toward you. It moves calmly and smoothly, glowing with joy. The closer to love you become, the better you can see love. What details do you notice that weren't visible when love was distant? The closer you come to love, the better you can feel love. What do you feel that you couldn't when barriers were in the way? The closer love comes, the better you can hear it. What sound does it make?

Love is now right in front of you, shining brightly. Are you ready to face love? Can you feel the warmth of love? What do you want to say to love? Say it. Speak your heart. Tell love your fears. Share your hopes and dreams with love. What does love say to you? Hear it.

Talk with love until your heart is empty of words. Love moves toward you. The glowing ball is as high as you are, and shines its lovelight fully on you. Reach for it with mind and heart. Step into the lovelight and let it illuminate and energize you, nurture and protect you. Love embraces you, enfolding you within itself so that you are filled and surrounded by love.

Within love is a gift. See, or sense, the gift of love. Notice details. Accept the gift.

Love's gift to you might be a heart-shaped valentine card. It's a gift of the heart, passionate red, yet romantic. The valentine is as big as you are. Reach out and bring it to you. Open it and read the sweet sentiments it bears, letting them fill your heart and mind. Hold the heart of love to your heart.

Love might be a sea, to show its changing tides and depths of emotion. Standing on the shore of the sea of love, water laps at your feet. As you gaze out over its expanse, the water is aquamarine, clear, and calm. It looks too enticing to resist, and so you dive in. The sea of love refreshes you as you swim, or you can just float and let love support you. All the bounty that the sea of love has to offer is yours.

As you're floating on your back in the sea of love, you hear the squeaks and clicks of a dolphin. The sounds become louder as the dolphin approaches, then there it is, nuzzling your ear with its beak. You drop your legs to face this creature who's so at home in the sea of emotion, and the dolphin swims into your arms. Together you swim, and dive, and frolic in love. The intelligence, playfulness, and communication skills of the dolphin, as well as its loyalty and protectiveness, reflect those of love.

Love might be a flower garden, a place that when lovingly tended produces an eyeful of colorful blossoms and a breathtaking array of scents. The garden might be in an open meadow, or protected by a wall with a gate in it. The aromas of the flowers reach you even before you enter the garden of love. Inhale delightedly, the collective aroma a soothing therapy for your psyche. Take a walk through the flowers. Some are short, barely brushing your ankles; others, like the lofty sunflowers, are almost as tall as you are. Stand proudly in the middle of your garden, surrounded by the myriad colors and forms of love. Feel safe and happy in your garden of love and, when weary, lie down and love will cushion you. Like varieties of flowers, the elements of love are uniquely designed, but each contributes the whole and enhances the garden of love.

Within love you might find a loving person. Is it a man or a woman? The person could be someone you know, or have known, who embodies the attributes of love that you value. Or it might even be a well-known person, a fictitious character, or an animal whom you relate to. It could be a spiritual being—either physical or nonphysical—whom you cherish.

Look into the loving eyes of the creature who stands before you. You are effortlessly drawn into an embrace. Feel strong arms enfolding you. Feel yourself wrapped in love. Feel yourself lifted in love. Feel yourself soar in love.

Your mind is full of the thought of love. Your heart is full of the feeling of love. Your body is full of the presence of love. When you love love, you become love.

By removing the barriers to love in your mind, you help remove the barriers to love in your life. The more you embrace love, the more love will embrace you. Feel empowered and protected by love. Be full of love. When you're able to love and be loved, you're truly love-able. You have been lovified!

Scaling Down

With your mind's eye, see or sense the scale you most often use to weigh yourself. See the style of it, the shape, and the color. Somewhere on the scale see printed or painted in bold letters a weight-loss slogan. It's brief and positive. It might be *Yes to Thin!* Or, *I Lose Weight Easily!* Or even just the word *YES!*

Once you have in mind the image of the scale with its slogan, enlarge it. Picture the scale twice as big, then double that. Make it so huge that the scale no longer fits in its usual spot.

Where to put this gigantic scale? Find a place for it in your mindscape. Make the place fun and bright so that you give your subconscious the message that losing weight can be enjoyable. Try putting the scale in the middle of a meadow filled with flowers, sunshine and birds. Or on a large flat rock shaped like a star, high on a cliff. See the scale in the center ring of a circus, with clowns and elephants all around. Wherever you put it, notice whether the air is warm or cool. What does it smell like? What sounds do you hear?

Above and behind the scale is a large square calendar pad of days. It's the kind of calendar that you peel off each page of to reveal a new day. The pad might be hanging from a tree, or suspended in mid-air, or stuck to the rump of an elephant. The top page shows today's day, date, and year. In what style and color are the letters and numbers printed?

You have now created the four main elements of your visualization: scale, slogan, environment, and calendar. See and sense them as clearly as possible. Reach out and touch them. Involve your senses. Hear the sounds. Smell the air. You're the number-one factor in any visualization, so be sure to put yourself in the picture.

Take off your shoes and step on the scale, feeling the coolness of it under your bare feet. As your current weight registers, a loud deep bell sounds. Look at the scale and see the number of pounds you weigh. Step off the scale and read your weight loss slogan again. Write your weight in large numbers across today's calendar page.

Now imagine that several of the calendar pages flutter and fly away as if blown off by a wind, the way early movies used to show the passage of time. When the pages stop blowing away, the date showing on the top page is two weeks from now. Across the page is written, in your handwriting, the number of pounds you want to weigh in two weeks.

Listen to your inner voice to make sure that the number you have set is realistic. If you hear your inner voice whining that you can't possibly lose that many pounds, reduce the number until you hear your inner voice agree that you can lose that weight in two weeks. Even if it's a small number, it's better to lose just one or two pounds than to be frustrated, then overeat, and end up gaining instead of losing. When the number you pick is realistic, you'll know, because you'll feel calm and confident in both your mind and your heart.

Once you feel comfortable with the number written across the calendar page, step onto the scale. The scale registers the exact same weight as the number written across the calendar page, and a slightly higher-toned bell rings. You're elated to have lost those pounds. A warm feeling of satisfaction fills you, bubbling up from your stomach to your head. You might raise your hand over your head in a triumphant gesture.

If the scale is in a meadow, you hear the birds and the flowers singing a little weight-loss ditty: "I love being thinner. Being thinner is a winner. Oh, how I love being thinner." If you're on a star-shaped rock, the rock is outlined in neon, which begins flashing. If you're standing in the center ring of the circus, the audience applauds, the clowns turn cartwheels, and the elephants trumpet approval. As you step off the scale, reading the slogan and feeling great about losing those pounds, the scale becomes smaller because you have become smaller.

Focusing again on the calendar, you see several more pages flutter and fly away in the wind. The date now on top is a month from now. What weight is written across the calendar page? Remember, make it realistic. How much weight do you believe you can lose in a month without placing your health at risk, or putting undue stress on yourself?

Before stepping on the scale, give yourself permission to have it register the same number of ·pounds as you've written across the calendar page. Read your slogan and step on the scale. A higher-toned bell rings. Again the number on the calendar and the number on the scale match. You're doing a downright, upright job of losing weight. Losing that extra poundage makes you feel wonderful both emotionally and physically. The birds and the flowers sing. The star-rock flashes. The circus audience applauds. Read your weight loss slogan and step off the scale. The scale becomes smaller, just as you're becoming smaller.

Picture future dates on the calendar pad in two-week or one-month increments, until you see your ideal weight written across the calendar page. As you allow the number on the calendar and the number on the scale to match, the tone of the bell that sounds becomes lighter because you're becoming lighter, and the scale becomes smaller because you're becoming smaller. How proud you are each time you achieve your goal! Join in the gleeful celebration of the birds, the flowers, the rock, the clowns, and the elephants.

Do this visualization daily for seven days to project your ideal weight to your subconscious. Then do it once a week, projecting ahead to next week's goal. When you actually step on your physical scale at the end of each week, give yourself permission for the number of pounds you weigh to match the number of pounds you visualized yourself weighing by that date.

Lightly Does It

Are you feeling heavy, sluggish, tense, or dim from eating too many negative foods, or thinking too many negative thoughts, or feeling too many negative emotions? Are there areas in your body that feel gooey, or places that feel as if they're blocked by a log jam? Here's an easy way to lighten up and get everything flowing smoothly.

First imagine that you're outdoors in a place that makes you feel strong and safe. In what environment do you see yourself? Standing barefoot on the earth, do you stand on soil, sand, or rock? Are your feet cushioned by leaves or moss? Do flowers or blades of grass tickle your ankles? Be aware of your weight on the soles of your feet pressing against the surface of the earth. Is the surface on which you stand dry or moist? Cool or warm? Yielding or hard? Smooth or gritty?

Once you feel "grounded," shift your attention to the top of your head. Imagine that a stream of light is pouring into your head from the sky above, or maybe someone is pouring light into your head from a pitcher that is never empty. What does the person who is helping you look like? What color and shape is the pitcher?

The light might tickle the top of your head as it begins to pour in. What color is the light? It might be a specific color, or white, or golden. Whatever the color, the light sparkles and dances as it arcs into the top of your head from the sky or the pitcher.

As you sense the light on top of your head, inhale it, pulling the light into you. You can imagine inhaling, or you can actually breathe air in through your nose, at the same time picturing light being sucked in from above. (Actually inhaling helps make what you're visualizing more real.) Allow the light to fill your head, feeling it sparkle and dance inside your skull effervescently.

Do you sense areas of your brain that are gooey with toxic thoughts, or dim with fear? The light absorbs all mental sludge and transmutes it into light, sparking your mind with new ideas. Even your ears, eyes, nose, and mouth light up. What does the light sound like? Look like? Smell like? What flavor is it?

The light flows merrily through your neck, out to your shoulders, then down your arms into your hands, clearing away all tension and stiffness in those areas. Feel the light tickling the very ends of your fingers. What does the light feel like? Is it smooth and silky, or dry and bubbly?

Now the light spills down into your chest, bathing your lungs and heart. Any dirt in your lungs, whether from smoking or the environment, is cleansed. Any emotional heaviness in your heart becomes light.

Exhaling, either literally or figuratively, push the light from your chest downward, past your belly button to where your thighs begin. If you feel areas of resistance where there are energy blocks, the light bursts right through them, clearing them away. Picture your entire trunk filled and surrounded with healing brightness, especially your digestive system. Light pours into your stomach, through the pyloric sphincter and the duodenum and into the small intestine. Sweet light fills and surrounds your pancreas, spleen, liver, gall bladder, kidneys, reproductive organs, and bladder.

When your trunk is full of merry, healthy light, let it cascade into your thighs. Feel it splash through your knees, slide between your calves and shins, and dance into your feet. Feel it tickle your toes.

If at any point you sense that the light is getting stuck in toxic goo or blocked in some way, that's your subconscious letting you know that that area needs extra attention. The places where the light jams up are often the same ones where fat jams up.

Wherever there are blockages, breathe light in from above, then exhale, putting your breath-light behind the blockage. Push against the blockage with gentle, steady pressure, or blow sharply. Take as many breaths as necessary to dissolve each barrier, so that light-energy can flow through your body unimpeded.

You're now filled with loving, laughing light from head to toe. Every nook and cranny of your body is touched by light. Each cell is kissed with light. Say (mentally or aloud), "Every cell in my body is healthy and happy with light." Say it again. "Every cell in my body is healthy and happy with light." And one more time. "Every cell in my body is healthy and happy with light."

Your body feels free and open, as if you had opened a window and allowed your body to fill with sunshine. You feel as light as a feather, as free as a bird, as sweet as a kiss. You glow like a star. Experiencing your body from the inside, it seems to feel smaller than when you looked at it from the outside. You feel invigorated. Your digestive system is stronger and more efficient. You hum with health.

Do this visualization whenever you're feeling heavy, sluggish, tense, or dim. If you're actually able to stand barefoot on the ground, it will add power to what you're visualizing. Because this is an enlightening experience, do it in the morning to energize yourself for the day ahead, or at night to clear yourself of the day's toxins, whether physical, mental, or emotional. If you're having an especially hectic day, or have eaten something you wish you hadn't, take a couple of minutes and visualize bright lovelight pouring through you from head to toe, cleansing and healing every part of your body.

Fat Out

To stop thinking fat and start thinking thin, it helps to get the word fat out of your mind. By getting rid of the word fat in your mind, you'll help get rid of the fat in your body.

Picture how the word *fat* might appear if it looked like what it means. The letters are fat, bulging into one another, and they're so weak that they have to lean on each other for support. There's nothing colorful about them, and nothing that sparkles. They seem pale and sickly looking. Dull.

What are the letters made of? Are they a sort of cheesy consistency? Or nutty? Or are they like greasy ground meat? Maybe the *f* is made out of cheese, the *a* is made out of pizza crust, and the *t* is two large French fries.

How do the letters move? Probably not too quickly, because their energy level is about on par with pudding. Maybe they scuffle and drag their feet. Or list to one side and so always go in circles. They might worm their way along slowly and laboriously, leaving a greasy trail behind them.

What sounds do the letters make as they move? Do they whine? Do they burp? Do they squish? Do they glug? Or do they wheeze?

The word *fat* is right in front of you. See, or sense, it as clearly as possible. Maybe a price tag hangs from one of the letters. A high price is written on it because you might be paying a high price for the extra fat you carry. The word *fat* is so large that it blocks your view of the future and gets in the way of your moving forward. It's difficult for you to have goals when you can't see them, and getting where you want to go can be exhausting. In short, *fat* impedes both your progress and your vision.

In addition, fat can sometimes prevent you from being close to people. They can't get close to you, and you can't get close to them because *fat* gets in the way.

Does *fat* make you angry? Have you had enough? Is it time to get rid of that *fat* so you can see what you want, and move toward it with ease? There's no time like the present, and the present is a gift, so get rid of that *fat* now.

How? First check to see if you have any attachments to fat. The attachments might take the form of ropes, strings, hooks, elastic bands, or black wires that stretch out from you and are tied or hooked to the letters. If you see that you are indeed holding onto *fat*, cut the ties that bind it to you. Use giant golden scissors, or a sword of silver, to cut your connections to *fat*.

When the attachments are severed, say no to *fat*. No, no, not like that. If it's a weak little no the *fat* won't budge an inch. Use your anger to say it like you mean it. NO! Fat moves back. Say it emphatically. NO!! *Fat* moves farther away and starts to sag. Shout it with feeling. NO! *Fat* turns paler, clearly frightened. NO!!! *Fat* starts to crumble and flatten out. Yell it with every fiber of your being. "N0-0-0-0-0!" *Fat* moves way back as if blasted by a strong wind.

Seeing *fat* on the run empowers you. With strength and surety you yell, "NO!! NO!! NO!! I don't want you! Get out of my mind! Get out of my body! Get out of my life! NO!!! NO!!! NO!!!" As you yell at *fat*, it's blasted farther and farther away. It becomes smaller and smaller until it's just a little blob of crumby dough. Then with one long and mighty, "NO-0-0-0-0-0-0-0-0-0!!!!!!!!," blast *fat* to smithereens. *Fat* is flat out gone.

Fat is out! Wowie, zowie, that feels great! You did it! Draw in a long, deep satisfied breath, and let it out with a feeling of pride and relief. Look around you. Nothing is in the way of being close to friends, or moving easily toward what you want. The way to increased success and happiness is clear.

Looking ahead, you see something bright glowing on the horizon. Curious, you move toward it. Your steps are quick and strong. Nothing blocks your way. The glow becomes bigger and brighter and seems to be moving toward you at the same time as you're moving toward it.

It's close enough now to make it out. It's the word *THIN*, looking like what it means. The letters are slim and strong, but flexible. What color are they? Pink because they're in the pink? Healthy, fresh green? Orange like a carrot? The color of flowers in the spring? Whatever color or colors the letters are, they look vibrantly healthy and glow with happiness.

What consistency are the letters? Crisp like celery? Woody like trees? Tender like fruit? Fibrous like flower stems? Soft like rose petals? Maybe the *T* is tall like a sapling that branches out at the top. The *H* is garlanded with flowers. The *I* is a sassy celery stalk. And the *N* is three bananas. Perhaps the *T* wears its heart on its head like a crown. The *H* has a crescent moon resting on its cross piece to signify a time of new beginnings. The *I* and the *N* both sport stars worn at rakish angles. Add whatever other details spark your mind and make you smile.

How do the *THIN* letters move? With verve and purpose, yet with a sense of grace and calm. Sometimes they're so energetic that they break into a little dance routine, or skip along, or turn cartwheels.

What sounds do the letters make as they move? Do they whistle a happy tune? Do they bubble with delight? Do they hum with power? Do they sing a merry *THIN* song?

We're thin, we're thin,
We're happy being thin!
We're thin, we win,
Hooray for being thin!
We're thin within,
We're happy being thin!

The *THIN* letters form a circle around you and do a celebration dance. Their enthusiasm is infectious, and you, too, dance in celebration. Then each letter embraces you. Delighted, you hug each letter in return. The *T* is in front of you, its heart on top. The *H* with its crescent moon is on your right. The *I* stands crisply behind you, its star twinkling. And the *N* stars to your left. You are surrounded and embraced by *THIN*, and with a happy heart you embrace *THIN* in return.

Then the *THIN* letters pick you up, lifting you over their heads in jubilation, and carry you wherever you want to go. The *THIN* letters are so active that they're never hanging around getting in your way. They don't block your view of the future, and they don't prevent you from getting where you want to go. In fact, they're a help instead of a hindrance. Their enthusiasm for life and their healthy glow is so attractive that they attract close friends and others who can help you achieve your goals. Whatever direction you choose to go in, *THIN* energy helps you get there more easily.

Looking into the future you see other bright, glowing balls of light on the horizon. Curious and excited about your future, you move toward the light. The *THIN* letters whistle and turn cartwheels. Hooray for *THIN*! Three cheers for you! *THIN* is in, and it suits you to a *T*.

Thin In

Losing the mental image of yourself as fat is as important as losing the actual pounds of fat. If you lose weight, and see a thinner you in the mirror, but your subconscious is seeing a mental picture of you looking fat, you could be headed for yo-yo land.

When you look thin in the mirror, but not in your mind, your subconscious will encourage you to overeat in order to regain the lost weight so that the mental image and the image in the mirror are the same. This occurs because one of the primary directives of the subconscious is consistency; the mental image and the physical image it sees must match. Here's a way to lose the mental image of yourself as fat, so you can lose pounds and keep them lost.

Imagine that you're walking in a meadow. Picture or sense the sun shining; feel it lying gently on your face and hands. The air smells of sun, earth, and flowers. Bees buzz busily from flower to colorful flower. Birds sing their songs to the wind. A breeze rustles the leaves of fruit trees and bushes at the edge of the meadow, where a sprawling orchard begins.

Feeling a little hungry, you saunter over to your favorite fruit tree. What kind is it? It might be an apple, banana, orange, mango, fig, or pear tree—each kind complete with a partridge. Or maybe your favorite fruit grows on a strawberry, blueberry, or raspberry bush. You espy two birds in the bush, and another one flies down from the sky and lands lightly in the palm of your hand, its heart beating quickly against your skin.

Pick the ripe fruit from the tree or bush and eat it. It's succulent and satisfies your appetite. Just beyond the tree or bush, you notice a high wall edging the orchard. In the wall are two large doors spaced widely apart. Both are closed. The door to your left has a sign that says OUT. The door to your right has a sign that says IN.

What do the doors look like? Are they the same design, or different? The door to the left might be old and scarred, with iron hinges. The door to the right might be arched and modern. Of what material are the doors made? Wood? Steel? Wrought iron? Glass? What color are they? What do the doorknobs look like? What shape are the keyholes?

When you have a good picture or sense of the doors, walk up to the one on the left, the OUT door. Looking above the door you see a plaque that says:

> *Whatever or whoever causes you strife,*
> *Passes through this door and out of your life.*
> *What goes out, stays out!*

Curious as to what this is all about, you try the doorknob. It turns easily. You give the door a slight push, and it swings out and away from you on squeaky hinges. Looking through the door you see trees. And more trees.

And some grass dotted here and there with flowers. And your favorite fruit. And birds. And more trees.

The bird in your hand, or the partridge in the tree, cocks its head, fixing you with one bright eye as if to say, "Okay, let's get on with it." Get on with what? Again you read the plaque above the door.

Whatever or whoever causes you strife,
Passes through this door and out of your life.
What goes out, stays out!

Suddenly you get it. You can get rid of whatever or whomever is in the way of you being healthy, thin, and happy, by pushing them out the OUT door. This could be fun.

You begin to think of the people who have disappointed, betrayed, humiliated, or harmed you. It might be just one person, or it might be several. It might be a parent, a relative, a teacher, a boss, a lover, or a friend.

As you think of each person, he or she appears in front of you, looking just as they did when they caused you strife. In no uncertain terms you tell each person to get out of your life. Say it like you mean it. "Get out of my life!" Say it with vigor. "Get out of my life!" Shout it enthusiastically. *"Get out of my life!"* Then push or kick each person through the open OUT door.

If you need help kicking them out of your life, simply visualize whatever help you need. If your abusers stubbornly resist, bring in a backhoe to dig them out and push them through the OUT door. Or bring in a crane to lift them out. Or bring in a giant crowbar to pry them out. Your favorite linebackers come to your aid. Or Batman.

Your anger, shame, and pain go out the OUT door with the people who've hurt you, or maybe you throw your negative emotions out separately. What do those emotions look like? Balls of fire? Rolls of barbed wire? Slime? Rusty nails? Shards of glass? Every bit goes out the OUT door.

Now picture *yourself* in front of you, at your fattest. When you see your fat self, you don't feel angry. In fact, you feel compassionate, because you know that it was the person or persons who hurt you with whom you were angry, not yourself. Shake hands with your fat self and ask if he or she has anything to say. Your fat self might tell you that he or she ate in order to absorb anger, shame, and pain. Or to fill the emptiness of not having the love you wanted and needed. Or to handle stress, contain panic, numb anxiety.

As you listen quietly to what your fat self tells you, awareness and forgiveness grow within your heart and mind. Filled with empathy, say that you understand, and give him or her a hug. Forgive your fat self for being fat. Then explain that you no longer want or need to be fat. Your fat self nods in agreement. You walk your fat self to the OUT door, and say goodbye. He or she steps out into the orchard and walks away, becoming lost among the trees. You close the OUT door.

You might feel a tinge of sadness in saying good-bye to your fat self, but mostly you feel glad. Whew! What a relief to lose all those heavy emotions, and people, and pounds. You feel lighter and clearer. A sense of accomplishment calms you and elates you at the same time. What a great feeling!

In the midst of feeling pleased, you remember the IN door. You run over and stand in front of it. It looks new and well maintained. The arch seems to signify that something or someone special will pass through it. You look up at the plaque in the arch over the door. It says:

Welcome in through this door
Everything you want—and more.
What comes in, stays in!

Excitedly you try the doorknob. It's locked. Darn! You try it again just to be sure. Nope. It jiggles, but it won't turn. Drat! What to do? Oh, woe.

Just before you succumb to disappointment, you notice that the bird has followed you over to the IN door. It's chirping and cocking its head at you, fixing you with one bright eye as if to say, "Okay, let's get on with it." You shake your head dejectedly. Again the bird seems to chirp, "Okay." Suddenly you realize that what the bird is really chirping is, "Oh, key."

Of course! You need a key to unlock the door so it will open to welcome in everything you want. The bird chirps, "Oh, key; oh, key," and points his beak in the direction of the key. The key might be hidden behind a brick in the wall. Or buried in the ground. It might be dangling from a branch of a tree on a ribbon. Or you might find the key in your pocket.

What shape is the key? How big is it? What's it made of? Feel the coolness of it against your skin. Heft it in your hand, feeling the weight. Your fingers clasp the shaft of the key, and you guide it into the keyhole. It fits perfectly. Give it a quick twist to the left, and hear the click of the lock opening.

Giving the IN door a gentle tug, it swings in toward you with ease and grace on well-oiled hinges. You look out the open IN door onto a lavish garden. A profusion of flowers of every kind and hue blankets the earth. Butterflies play among the petals. Fruit trees and money trees dot the landscape, their branches weighted with their offerings. Flocks of doves and gaily colored parrots swoop through the sky. The landscape is so rich, so lovely, that you stand there for a moment, feasting your eyes.

Standing under the tree looking out, you begin to think about what you want. You want to be thin. No sooner does the thought illuminate your mind than you see your thin self walking toward the IN door. Your thin self moves easily and wears stylish new clothes. Smiling broadly, you welcome in your thin self. He or she smiles in return and steps lightly across the threshold, coming in the IN door. Thin is in.

You shake your thin self's hand, and maybe give him or her a hug. Your arms go easily around your thin self, and beneath your hands his or her body feels slim and fit. You express how glad you are to have your thin self in your life. Your thin self's eyes shine, and he or she nods, saying how good it feels to be here.

Your thin self then holds out a hand to you, palm up. A small and precious gift lies there. A gift to give you confidence and strength. What is it? With gratitude you accept the gift, and give your thin self a gift in return. What is it?

Once you've welcomed your thin self in through the IN door and into your life, the two of you begin to talk excitedly about all the things you're going to be able to do and experience. The clothes you'll be able to wear. The compliments you'll receive. The people you'll meet. The places you'll go. With much joy you and your thin self celebrate how happy you are to be slim and healthy.

Your thin self reminds you that whatever else you want, all you have to do is think it and see it to get it. Whatever or whomever you think you want will come in the IN door and into your life. What a great feeling!

To prevent anyone (your fat self, for instance) or anything you don't want from coming in, picture a big bright ball of light filling and surrounding the IN doorway. Light keeps darkness away. Or have a doorperson stationed just outside the IN door to keep out the uninvited.

This is an excellent visualization to do often when you first start dieting in order to align your inner image with your outer goal. Then do it maybe once a week for reinforcement. If your fat self tries to reassert itself, simply escort *fat* out the OUT door, and welcome *thin* in the IN door.

Less Stress

The nervous energy of stress can make you want to overeat unless you do something to relax. If your schedule is ultra busy, manage stress by doing a relaxing visualization. Reducing tension through visualization can be done more easily and quickly than doing a relaxing physical activity, yet it's effective because your subconscious responds to mental images and feelings the same way it does to physical images and feelings.

Picture your favorite bathtub. It might be the one at home, or at a hotel you stayed in, or a tub you saw pictured in a magazine. It might be indoors or outdoors. It could be a fantasy tub located outdoors on a deserted tropical island with a view of a serene blue sea surrounded by lush foliage and brilliantly colored flowers.

See your tub exactly the way you want it. What is your tub made of? Porcelain, fiberglass, metal, wood, tile, or stone? What color is it? What shape is it? Make it big enough and deep enough to accommodate you.

What does the surrounding area look like? What color and material are the walls? Does a soft thick carpet cover the floor or ground? See a pile of soft thick towels monogrammed with your initials resting on a corner of the tub. Next to your favorite soap is a large natural sponge.

Would you like a rubber ducky? See or sense details clearly in order to make the scene as real as possible.

Hanging from a door hook, a tree branch, or a statue's hand is the bathrobe you always wear. Get out of the clothes you're wearing, and put your robe on. Then turn on the faucets to fill your tub with water. Put your hand under the spigot to feel the temperature of the water, adjusting until it's just right. The water is whatever color you want: sea blue, champagne gold, strawberry pink, or peach.

On a shelf above the tub is a selection of wonderful things you can add to your bath to enhance it. *Joy* bubble bath. A box of *Weight Cleanse* bath salts. A bottle labeled *Less Stress Oil. Love* bath beads. Hmmmm. What to put in? What the hey—add them all to the bath water.

When the tub is filled, slip out of your robe and get in, holding onto something so you don't slip. The water is exactly the temperature you like, and it feels silky against your skin. Stretch out the full length of the tub, resting your head on a special tub pillow, and close your eyes contentedly.

The water covers you completely, making you feel deliciously warm and safe. It soaks away pain, both physical and emotional. Tightly coiled springs of stress unwind. Knots in muscles loosen. Anxiety is bathed away. Let the aromas of the bath oils and beads soothe your mind. Anger is extinguished. Dis-ease is eased in the water's warmth. Fat melts. Stress is soothed. Worries evaporate. Your mind and body feel relaxingly fluid.

Soak in the tub for as long as you want. A few minutes before you're ready to get out, wash yourself with the large natural sponge. It feels soft but invigorating against your skin, and it stimulates your circulation. Gently rub your body, paying loving attention to the areas where you especially want to release tension or fat. Use the sponge to absorb fat as it melts, sucking it up so you don't have to suck it in.

As you scrub off emotional grime, your mind and body feel clean. As you wash away physical tension, your body feels smooth. As you are cleansed of unwanted fat, your body feels lighter.

When you've bathed for as long as you want, get out of the tub. Pluck a soft, thick towel from the pile and dry yourself. Rub off any last drops of stress. Wipe off tension. When you reach for your robe you find a brand-new one in the style and color you like most. Slip it on and feel enfolded in soft serenity.

When you turn back to the tub to pull the plug, you notice that the water is gray, clouded with the tension, worry, and fat that you have washed off. The more negativity that was soaked out, the darker the water is. Squeeze worry, fat, and tension out of the sponge and rinse it in clear water. Pull the plug and watch the water, dirty with physical and emotional toxins, go down the drain. Hear the sound the water makes as it flows out of the tub.

As the water drains, you feel as if all tension has completely drained from your body. Your body feels clear and light. Your mind feels clear and bright. With calm and strength, you're ready for life.

Number 1

Do you look larger than you feel? Do you look round and full on the outside, while inside you feel flat and empty? Looking like something, but feeling like nothing—*nada, rien,* zero, zilch, zip—isn't fun. It also isn't healthy or helpful. If you look and feel like a *0*, it's time for a change.

In order to effect change it's important to first acknowledge what it is that's about to be changed. Understanding what's to be changed helps you want to make the change. By acknowledging that the shape of your body doesn't suit you, and that it makes you uncomfortable, you give yourself direction and motivation for changing it.

Understanding why you want to change your body can take great courage and honesty. If you want extra strength for this visualization, go to your Palace of Power and infuse yourself with whatever energy you need to proceed.

Begin by imagining yourself as a round rubber ball. (A *0* is just a two-dimensional slice of a three-dimensional ball.) How big are you? What color is the rubber? How thick is it? Thin and flexible like the skin of a beach ball? Thick and hard like a rubber handball?

Ask yourself what effect being a rubber ball has on you. Does the thickness of the rubber separate and distance you from others? Does it make it more difficult to realize your dreams? Does being round make you less stable? Do you feel tossed around by people in particular and life in general? Are you hit more often than you're up at bat? Is it hard to stop when you want to?

Sometimes you can throw your weight around, but people may often try to push you around. And it can take only a nudge from someone to start you rolling downhill. Pretty soon you're rolling downhill faster and faster, and you can't stop. You're out of control. The more momentum you gain, the more you panic, and you have to crash in order to stop. Or you hit bottom.

Now ask yourself what purpose being a rubber ball serves. Does it make you look more substantial than you actually feel? Do you look large to compensate for feeling small? Do you believe that bigger is better because it lets you throw your weight around?

Does the rubber insulate you against hurt? Do you use pain and anger to make the rubber thicker and harder in order to keep from being punctured and deflated? Is it a repository for negative thoughts and feelings? Do you hope that if you're round and fat as you were as a baby, when you were protected and nurtured, that you'll receive the same attention now?

When someone or something in your life throws you, does being round and rubbery keep you from being hurt? Does the rubber help you bounce back from dropping out of life? Is it a scapegoat for your unhappiness? Does it make you feel more whole?

If you answered yes to even one of the above questions, it's worth changing your shape. Begin by filling the emptiness inside you. First picture a large empty glass in front of you. What shape is it? It might be tall and straight, it might be round, or it might be a champagne glass. It's clear, but it could have some color to it. Your initials are etched into the glass.

Having bravely and honestly acknowledged the things that make you uncomfortable with yourself, it's time to acknowledge the things that make you comfortable; an assessment that in its own way requires just as much courage and candor. By consciously recognizing your positive qualities and honoring positive deeds, you can fill the empty glass with love. You're not being egotistical because you're not comparing yourself to others and finding yourself less than, or better than. This is simply observing what is of value about you, and ingesting it to fill the void.

The first positive quality you might want to recognize is that of being open to changing the shape of your body. As you acknowledge that you *are* open to the possibility (or you wouldn't be reading this visualization), love nectar appears in the bottom of the glass. It looks delicious. What color is it? Does it look thick like honey or thin like milk? How much is there?

If you feel pangs of hunger when you see it, drink up, even if it's only a swallow. Feel the love nectar glide across your tongue. Or maybe it dances. What does it taste like? Sweet? Minty? Tart? What temperature is it? Hot? Cold? Warm? Cool? What texture is it? Smooth like honey? Bubbly like mineral water? Now let it slide down your throat and begin to fill the emptiness inside.

A recent deed to honor is your willingness to look at the things about being fat that make you uncomfortable. As you acknowledge that indeed it took courage and honesty to answer those questions, more love nectar appears in the bottom of the glass. You can drink it up, or if you prefer, leave it in the glass so you can add to it.

What do you *like* about your body? Do you have nice eyes? Is your smile friendly? Do you have healthy hair? Are your teeth strong? Are you dexterous with your hands? Is your skin smooth? Are you coordinated? Do you have fast reflexes?

What qualities do you like about yourself? Are you kind? Smart? Honest? Strong? Gentle? Generous? Responsible? Empathetic? Considerate? Witty? Zany? Helpful? Dependable? Easy-going? Organized? Punctual? Tidy? Creative? Do you like to laugh? Do you have a good memory?

What did you do yesterday, or the day before, or the day before that, that made you feel good about yourself? Did you feed a stray cat or remember a friend's birthday? Or pass on that piece of pie? Hold the door open for someone? Send flowers to someone who was sick? Wash the dishes in the sink? Drive safely? Eat or drink something healthy? Smile at someone? Do you generally try to help friends? Do you take care of the tasks for which you're responsible? Do you try to do your best?

For each characteristic, quality, and deed that you value about yourself, whether little or large, see the level of love nectar rise higher and higher in the glass. When the glass is full, lift it, feeling the weight and substance of love, and drink every drop. Feel the love nectar glide across your tongue and slide down your throat. Taste it. Enjoy it. Loving yourself can be a delicious experience.

Just as the level of love rose in the glass as you acknowledged what is positive about yourself, see the love nectar filling the emptiness within you. Feel it pouring in. The more you value yourself, the less emptiness there is. The hunger pangs disappear. By recognizing the positive, you eliminate the negative.

As you drink in love and the hole inside you fills, a curious thing happens. The outside of you loses its roundness. You begin to narrow and straighten. The thick rubber shell becomes thin because you don't need the insulation; your love for yourself protects you. By valuing yourself, you don't have to be large to feel big.

You like how this feels. You stand straighter. You feel more stable and in control. It's going to be hard for anyone to push you around now. You stand taller. Life looks better and more interesting. You feel optimistic about the future. You realize that you can protect and nurture yourself. You stand proud.

If you still feel a little empty, think of more things you respect about yourself, and fill another glass with love. Sometimes just one acknowledgment can fill the whole glass. Drink it up so it goes down into you and fills you. Drink as many glasses of love as you need to fill the hole. When you're full of love and no longer feel like nothing, *nada, rien,* zero, zip, zilch, then you're really something! You're not a *0,* you're numero uno, number 1.

Whenever you start to feel round and empty, take a minute to review your positive characteristics, qualities, and deeds. Drink them in, fill up, and be number 1. Make the hole whole.

Control Central

Picture the inside of your brain looking like the center of operations inside a spaceship that's traveling at the speed of thought. Control central might be brain-shaped, or look like two gigantic pie pans, one upside-down on top of the other. Along the round walls and ceiling are control panels with flashing lights. Banks of computer screens display constantly updated information from outside and inside your body.

The name of the ship is your name, displayed in lights on the floor or ceiling. The basic decor is done in white, gray, and cream colors, with energy supplied through red wires. In the center is a column of cables leading down through a hole in the floor, relaying information from your brain to your body, and from your body to your brain.

Computers that process data, numbers, words, and time are arranged on the left side of the space in a linear and logical manner. Words and numbers flash on the screen. There's a steady hum of activity and clicks of data registering.

On the right is a hodgepodge of holograms projecting three dimensional scenes of your environment, interior and exterior shots of your body, faces of people, memories, dreams, paintings, and dances. The right side is a hubbub of music and tones.

On each side of your brain, in front of an oval-shaped porthole, is a command chair in blue, green, gray, brown, or hazel. What color, size, shape, and style is each chair? Sitting in the chair on the left side is a man. Sitting in the chair on the right is a woman. These are your Mind Mates. Each one looks out through a porthole and switches the data coming in to either the left or right side of your brain. Each Mind Mate also has access to data from the interior, again sorted to the left or right.

As the captain of your ship you decide to get some information about weight control. You approach the man in the chair on the left and take a peek out the porthole. You see your present surroundings and know the names of the objects you see, and how many there are.

The Mind Mate on the left is wearing a streamlined, wear-resistant uniform. He's extremely busy overseeing the processing of data and doesn't realize that you've come up on the bridge. Get his attention by clapping your hands, or shouting "Yo" or "Hey." What color are his hair and eyes? How old is he? How tall? How much does he weigh? Does he have a name?

As soon as you command his attention, tell him to punch up all data on weight. He keys in the word *Weight*, and information starts flashing up on the screen. First, the Webster's Dictionary definition of weight: "the amount that a thing weighs." Second, the number of pounds you weigh, with a notation that you are a person, not a thing. After your current weight, your ideal weight has been computed according to your gender, age, height, bone structure, and activity level. The number of calories needed per day to maintain your current weight is computed by multiplying the number of pounds you weigh by fifteen calories.

The next batch of information is about weight-loss programs. The man in the chair might tell you, "We're not showing any weight-loss programs listed." Or, "The operating weight program is Fat: I eat whatever I want, whenever I want, wherever I want, and evermore than I need."

The next batch of data lists your beliefs about weight. When they flash on the screen you're surprised to see that they're in your handwriting. Some of the beliefs might be:

- Diets don't work.
- I can never lose weight.
- Losing weight is difficult.
- I gain back twice as much as I lose.
- Exercise makes me eat.
- I am worthless.
- I deserve to be fat.
- I am a bad person.
- I should be punished.
- I can't handle stress.
- I can't control my eating.
- I hate the past.
- I am afraid of the future.
- Life is overwhelming.
- I am helpless.
- I am powerless.
- I don't like myself.

After seeing the data, it's clear that your brain is thinking fat. Instruct the man in the chair to erase all fat thoughts and beliefs from the data banks. He keys in *fat* and hits delete. Blip. All fat thoughts, programs, and beliefs are deleted. The screen displays the information: Fat Deleted. Then it instructs: Think Healthy Ideas Now.

Issue new instructions. Tell your Mind Mate the ideal weight you've decided on. He types in the number of pounds. See that number fill the screen. Ask him to compute the number of calories you need a day in order to lose a pound a week. See that number on the screen. For the operating weight program, he types in "Thin: I eat whatever I want, whenever I want, wherever I want, and I stop before I'm full."

Write your Think Healthy beliefs now, using an electronic pen to write directly on the computer screen in your handwriting.

- Diets always work.
- I lose weight easily.
- Lost weight stays lost.
- Exercise is satisfying.
- I am valuable.
- I deserve to be my ideal weight.
- I am a good person.
- I forgive myself my mistakes.
- I handle stress well.
- I control my eating effortlessly.
- I am at peace with the past.
- I look forward to the future.

- Life is an adventure.
- I am powerful.
- I love myself every day, in every way.

Feel the positive energy of your Think Thin program begin to flow into every part of your mind, body, and life. Then walk over to the right side of your brain to talk to the woman. Sneak a peek out the right porthole. You recognize the objects and people in your present environment, and can estimate their distance from you and from each other. You especially notice motion and esthetic touches.

The Mind Mate on the right sensed your arrival and is already waiting for you, prepared to share the information you desire. She's wearing light that twirls and dances around her body to its own light music. What color are her hair and eyes? Does she have a name? She knows yours and greets you warmly. What does the pitch and tone of her voice sound like? She exudes a sense of playfulness, spontaneity, and sensuality.

The woman takes you by the hand, and, without moving through time or space, you're in front of a hologram that projects you being fat. In the hologram you might look angry, frightened, and sad all at the same time. The environment around you looks dark and scraggly, lifeless.

The woman looks questioningly at you. You shake your head no. She touches her hand to the hologram, and *blip-ity, blob-ity, blip*, the fat you disappears and is replaced with an image of you at your ideal weight. You look at peace with yourself and the world. Your environment is bright and lush. Again the woman looks at you questioningly; you nod.

The woman, with one hand still touching the hologram, touches you with her other hand, and in the blink of a thought you're inside the hologram. You're standing in that bright, lush environment at your ideal weight. Look down at your feet. What are you wearing on them? Feel how differently your feet feel when you're standing on them at your ideal weight.

Look around your ideal weight environment. Whatever you think you want in it appears in the blink of a thought. Likewise, whomever you think you want in your life arrives. Make your ideal weight world just the way you want it. Be and do whatever you want.

Picture Control Central whenever you want to be in a good frame of mind about losing weight. Don't be left out. When you're in your right mind, you think thin!

Burning Calories

Mental exercise done in conjunction with physical exercise helps align body and mind. When you visualize calories burning, you increase the calorie-burning efficiency of your body, because the body responds to what the mind is thinking. This was demonstrated in tests done by physiologist Edmund Jacobson in the 1920s. He attached electrodes to supine subjects and instructed them to visualize themselves running, and the muscles associated with running contracted.

When you show your subconscious pictures of how you want your body to look and function, your body will get with the program. If you want your body to burn calories efficiently, here's a way to get that image across to your subconscious.

Begin by picturing a fire burning somewhere in your body, but not harming you in any way. You might sense a fire in a central area of your body such as your stomach, your chest, or your head. Or you might have a fire in your belly with flames that reach up to your heart and your mind so that all three are ignited with the same goal.

In what type of environment is the fire burning? A fireplace? An incinerator? An open hearth? A clearing in the woods? A garbage dump? On a beach? Or on a rocky cliff? Be sure to practice safe burning by containing the fire.

How big is the fire? Your subconscious might let you know how high or low your metabolism is by the size of the fire you see. If the fire would barely melt ice, it certainly won't be able to burn calories. You have the power to control the fire's size, so make it blaze. See the flickering red, white, orange, yellow, and blue flames. Feel how the fire warms your body. Make the fire roar. Hear it snap and crackle. As you concentrate on the fire in your body, you may actually sense heat.

The fire can represent your burning desire to lose weight. Or it might just be pure energy. Or enthusiasm for life. Or unpleasant emotions put to good use. Use the emotions from an experience in the past that was a "trial by fire." Or have fire represent the burning anger you feel toward others, or even toward yourself.

When your fire is burning brightly, it's time to burn those calories. What do the calories look like? They might look like little charcoal briquettes. Or logs. Or globules of fat. Or bubbles of gas. Or wads of paper. The only requisite is that the calories are plentiful and flammable. Dietitians estimate that it takes about 15 calories a day to maintain each pound of weight. By burning 500 calories a day more than you take in, you can lose a pound a week.

How many calories does each briquette, or log, or bubble, equal? Throw the calories on the fire. Do it one by one by hand, or use a shovel. Or have Campfire Girls or Boy Scouts tend the fire, gathering calories and feeding them into the fire. Or create a Cal Pal who directs calories into the fire. Or the calories could simply flow into the fire of their own accord.

Feeding the fire with calories makes the fire burn bigger and brighter. Hear the hiss and crackle of the calories burning. The calories glow briefly, then turn to ash and disappear in the heat of the flames. The calories burn quickly and cleanly, leaving no residue. Feel the heat produced by the burning calories.

As the calories burn, your body feels like a steam engine, burning fuel to create power to take action. Your center of gravity, just below your belly button, feels centered and strong. Your heart feels cleared of negative emotions and alive with passion for life. Your mind feels bright and clear, ready to accomplish goals and solve problems. Your whole being feels charged with energy.

Seeing between five hundred and a thousand calories burning every day will encourage your body to burn calories more efficiently. Doing this mental visualization before, or during, physical exercise—whether walking briskly, working out, or playing racquetball—will increase the calorie-burning benefits of the exercise.

Love Food

What have you been feeding your heart and mind? Left-over feelings? Stale ideas? Frozen frustration? Half-baked dreams? If your heart and mind are hungry for something fresh and nourishing, here's a recipe for hearty love food.

First decide where you want to enjoy your love meal, creating a mental image, or sense, of the environment. Do you want to eat at home, in your favorite restaurant, or some special spot outdoors? What size and shape is the table? Does it have placemats or a tablecloth? Candles? Flowers? What design is the chair?

What does the place setting look like? Are you going to use silverware or goldware? What color is the plate? Is it china or ceramic? Does it have a design on it? Maybe good-luck symbols are scattered across it, or your initials are intertwined with hearts, or flowers, or stars. Around the rim of the plate, written in gaily colored letters, is your positive slogan: "I am nourished by love." Or, "I am filled with love and light." Or, "love energizes me."

Now picture, or sense, your stove at home. On the burners are pots and pans in which love food is cooking. The pots have lids on them, but the aromas that escape and curl into your nostrils are tantalizing. Something is baking in the oven and smells delicious.

Who's doing the cooking? It might be you, or some-one else. It could be someone you know: mother, father, friend, lovemate. Or it could be someone you don't know: your fairy godmother, Wolfgang Puck, Mary Poppins, or Winnie the Pooh. Create whomever you want to cook love food for you. Have one cook, or several, each one con-tributing their speciality.

Take your plate with your personal slogan around the rim and, holding it in one hand, or setting it down next to the stove, begin to serve yourself your love meal. Lift the lid on the pan nearest to you. Inside is love. Does it simmer or sizzle? What color is love? What shape? Help yourself to a big hunk of love. If you're really hungry, take two or three pieces—you can have as much love as you want without gaining an ounce. Put a generous ser-ving of love on your plate.

Lifting the lid on the next pot, you discover opti-mism. Optimism might look like fresh yellow corn, or maybe pink peas. Spoon a heaping portion of optimism onto your plate next to the love.

In the third pot vitality tea is bubbling briskly. Is it clear like light? Golden like honey? Red like a hibiscus flower? Pour it into the cup or mug that matches your plate.

Baking in the oven is enthusiasm bread. Cut yourself a thick slice. Is it white bread, or whole grain? Does it have nuts, or maybe heart-shaped raisins? Put the bread on your plate.

Is there anything else you need or want to make your love meal complete? A sauce of light for the love, perhaps? A dollop of open-minded jam for the bread? A vivacious condiment? A spoonful of elation to sweeten the tea?

Carry your full plate and brimming cup to where you have chosen to eat, and set them down on the table. Sit down and enjoy your love meal. This can be a special dinner just for you, or you can invite someone to share your love with, or even have a dinner party.

The love is so tender you can cut it with your fork. It's warm and smooth in your mouth and seems to melt. What flavor is Love? Eat some Optimism. Drink some Vitality. Take a few bites of Enthusiasm.

Love food nourishes feelings, freshens ideas, and enriches dreams. Eat all the love food you want, whenever you want; it's nonfattening and nourishes the good feelings you have for yourself.

New View

Being able to see yourself can be a challenge, but it's necessary in order to change the old into the new. Here's a way to make seeing a new view of yourself fun and easy.

Imagine that you're outside the house or apartment where you live. See the form and color of the structure. Of what material is it made? What kind of roof does it have? What does the landscaping look like? Where are the cars parked?

When you can see, or sense, where you live from several angles, go to a window and look in. If the window is on an upper floor, simply float up to it and stand on air, or hover in front of it. If it's daytime, sunshine fills the room. If it's nighttime, the room is illuminated with bright lights.

See yourself at home being thin. Does the interior of your home look the same, or has your thin self made changes in the decor? What are you doing? You might be doing some of the same things as when you were overweight, or you might be doing different things. Or you might be doing the same things differently.

One thing is for sure: you look different. Take a good look at yourself doing whatever you're doing, whether it's talking on the phone with a friend, taking care of some business, cooking, watching television, or reading. The clothes you're wearing are new and flatter your slim body. What color are the clothes? What style? Does the material have a special design?

Check out your body. It looks fit and lithe, and you look happy being in it. There's a smile on your face, and your eyes have a warm light in them. Your hair shines with health. Have you changed your hair color, or is it the same? What about you has stayed the same? What do you notice that's different? It might be how you look, the way you move, or even how you talk.

See yourself engaged in different activities at home. When you're talking on the phone your face is animated with the enjoyment of sharing with a friend. When you're taking care of business details, you concentrate with pleasure, your motions efficient and effective. When you're in the kitchen, see yourself cooking up healthy food. When you're watching television, reading, or listening to music, your body appears fluidly relaxed. See yourself bathing. Your arms, legs, chest, and stomach are well shaped, and the lines of your body flow in strong curves that are pleasing to the eye.

Seeing yourself thin and happy is immensely satisfying. You like this new view of yourself. Feeling proud, you raise a victorious fist to the sky. Or maybe you do a victory dance, taking a triumphant twirl. In fact, you look so good to yourself, so attractively healthy that you can't wait to congratulate yourself.

Picture yourself standing in front of your front door. What is the color and design of the door to where you live? You're carrying a bottle of sparkling cider in one hand, and holding a bunch of colorful helium-filled balloons in the other. With both hands full, how are you going to knock on the door or push the buzzer? Try tapping the door with your foot, or using your elbow to push the buzzer.

The door opens and your thin self is standing there smiling at you. Give him or her a big smile in return. What is your thin self wearing? Your thin self opens the door wider, and tells you to please come in. You hand him or her the bottle of sparkling cider and the balloons. Your thin self is delighted to receive them. You're so glad to see your thin self that you give him or her a huge hug. Notice how supple and strong your thin body is to hug.

In the living room, your thin self lets the balloons go. They float up to the ceiling and bob around up there, the ribbons trailing down like party streamers. He or she goes into the kitchen and comes back with two champagne glasses for the sparkling cider.

You and your thin self sit together on the sofa and drink a toast to being thin, fit, and fabulous. "Here's to thin. Congratulations. May thinness endure in health and happiness. Three cheers for thin!"

A curious thing happens as your selves are sitting next to each other, toasting being thin and talking intimately about the positive changes that being thin has brought about. Without thought or effort you slide closer and closer to your thin self. You're sitting shoulder to shoulder, hip to hip, and knee to knee. Suddenly, *whoosh!* You're no longer sitting next to your thin self, you're sliding right into thin. *Schwillpp*—you *are* your thin self. Look at your hands. Look down at your feet on the floor. Touch your heart. Put your hand to your head. Feel your stomach. Sure enough—you *are* thin!

You look around the living room in your home. No one is there but thin you. You look down at the sofa seat where your fat self was sitting. There's nothing there but a peculiar-looking mound of something. It's the fat that was left over when you slid into thin; the fat that wouldn't fit in your thin body. The size of the mound depends on how much extra fat there was to lose. Get a broom, a shovel, or a vacuum cleaner, and clean up the mound of fat. Where do you dispose of it?

After you've cleaned up, pull a balloon down from the ceiling and write a wish on it with a felt tip marker. You can have as many wishes as there are balloons. (And then you can visualize another bunch of balloons, and another, and another—) They can be wishes about being thin, or any other aspect of your life. See the words in your handwriting on the surface of each colored balloon.

Holding the ribbons to make a bouquet of balloons, take them over to the window you were looking into, and open it. Look out, seeing the view you normally see from that window. Then, one by one, set the balloons free, watching as they carry your wishes up to the sky. There they will come true and come back to find you on the brightly colored ribbons of your dreams. One wish has already come true. You are thin!

Light as a Feather

If you're feeling heavy in heart, mind, or body, here's a way to lighten up. Imagine yourself in a place outdoors in which you can feel safe, yet free. It can be near your Palace of Power, or anywhere on the planet, real or imagined.

Bring the elements of your special place into focus. What does the ground look like? Is it earth or sand? Is it covered with grass, leaves, pine needles, or moss? Take off your shoes and feel the ground with your bare feet. Are there rocks nearby, or trees, or water? Are there flowers and fruit trees? What temperature is the air? Warm or cool? Is it humid or dry? What scents does the air carry to your nose? What sounds does the air carry to your ears? Taste something. Pick a fruit and eat it, or drink some water.

When you have created an outdoor environment that makes you feel both safe and free, sit down in the middle of it. You might sit cross-legged on the ground, or you might create a sofa to sit on, or a throne. A feeling of expectancy sparkles in the air, as if something or someone special were going to arrive. From behind an outcropping of rock, or from behind a tree, or from behind the curtain of a waterfall, steps a Native American medicine man.

How is he dressed? What is he wearing on his feet? How tall is he? From his shiny black hair hangs a large eagle feather, and in his hand he holds another, even larger, feather. Notice the shape and color of the feather in his hand. His shining black eyes are like deep pools of wisdom, lit with compassion. His bearing conveys quiet strength and power.

The medicine man walks over and stands before you. He introduces himself. What does his voice sound like? Hear who he is, and what his name is. He asks how he can help you. Tell him that you feel heavy and would like to feel light. He nods, sagely, then begins gathering natural materials from the ground and shaping it into a bed.

With a wave of the feather in his hand, the medicine man invites you to lie down on the bed of leaves, pine needles, flowers, moss, or sand that he has fashioned for you. You do so, and immediately feel fresh, organic energy flowing into your body, soothing it and strengthening it.

The medicine man sits cross-legged by your side, midway between your head and feet at about your waist. Slowly and reverently he opens the medicine pouch that hangs from a thong around his neck. As he takes a pinch of power powder from the pouch and sprinkles it on the feather in his hand, he talks to you.

How does he address you? He might call you by your name, or address you as Child or Granddaughter. He might call you Little One, or an Indian name. He suggests that some of your heaviness might come from thinking heavy thoughts. That perhaps you think of yourself as heavy, and also that many of your thoughts are weighed down with negativity.

Holding the long feather lightly in his hand, the medicine man touches the crown of your head and your forehead with it. Then using short outward strokes all around your head, he brushes away negative thoughts. Your mind clears and lightens. If you had a headache, it's brushed away. Your mind becomes calm, yet at the same time your thoughts become brighter. With peace of mind, you close your eyes.

The medicine man next touches the power feather to your heavy heart, suggesting that the emotional ties that really bind are those of anger. He understands that sometimes a situation makes one feel helpless, and that anger restores a sense of power. But whether angry with others, or with yourself, anger constricts the flow of love. Anger can also create fat. Angry energy that isn't expressed or released needs somewhere to go, so it goes to fat. Once there, anger binds it to your body.

The words are spoken with compassion, and the insights you gain help heal the anger. As the feather touches your chest, you feel the bonds of anger around your heart loosen. Your heart expands, allowing love to flow freely throughout your body.

As your body becomes invigorated with the energy of love, you become aware of tightness around certain parts of your body, as if something were tied tightly around them. You open your eyes and are surprised to see people whom you're angry with tied to different parts of your body. They could be parents, siblings, teachers, friends, ex-lovers, bosses, coworkers, etc. How do they look? They might look like dark storm clouds with faces, or they might look like the actual people. Even though your anger with them may be justified, it keeps them attached to you.

Notice which people are attached to which areas of your body, and by what. Some might be attached by black string or rope, others by thick cables and chains. Many of the places to which they're tied are areas where your body holds onto fat: waist, stomach, hips, and thighs, and so on.

See who's attached to your chest, constricting love; to your throat, inhibiting expression; to your mouth, blocking nourishment; to your nose, suffocating you; to your ears, deafening you; to your eyes, blinding you; to your back, making you bend; to your hands, preventing you from reaching for what you want; to your ankles, shackling your progress. Seeing the connection between a particular person and a particular area of your body will provide insight about the effects of your relationship with that person.

The ropes and chains of anger that shackle you to people are short, so the more people with whom you're angry, the more crowded it will be around you. The people attached to you by anger can prevent those you love, or who love you, from getting close to you. Anger isolates, inhibits, and blocks you.

The medicine man, however, has the power to get close to you no matter who or what is in the way, and you see him still sitting cross-legged by your side. Using sharp strokes, he passes the feather across your face, neck, shoulders, chest, sides, waist, stomach, groin, legs, and feet. Like a sword, the power feather cuts the fetters of anger, releasing them. *Pop!* The bonds break. *Pop!* The cords snap off. *Pop!* The chains burst apart.

Sense the tension break. Feel the anger being released. You are free of the people who were bound to you, and they, too, are freed. Your body, mind, and heart feel free and light as if they've been let out of prison. Fat loses its hold on you and is brushed away by the power feather.

The medicine man knows that anger often masks pain, and that fat can be a repository for pain as well as anger. He again touches the feather to the crown of your head and to your forehead. Then he leans over you and blows sharply into the middle of your forehead, expelling the pain from painful memories. You can have the memories if you want, but you don't need the pain.

Again he touches your heart with the power feather. He leans over you, and with utmost tenderness reaches into your heart and pulls out the black stone of pain that weighs you down. Holding the stone in one hand, he taps it with the power feather. The stone turns white. He tosses the stone up into the air, and it turns into a dove and flies away. You breathe deeply and freely.

Once more the medicine man brushes your body with the feather, from head to toe, sweeping away woe. He sweeps away the pain of broken dreams and of not enough love. As disappointments, resentments, and fears are swept from you, they no longer need fat to hold them, so the fat is swept away, too. No pain, no gain.

Lying there while the medicine man heals you of anger and pain, you look gratefully into the pools of wisdom that are his eyes. You thank him from the depths of your mind and heart. He acknowledges your gratitude with a smile and a nod.

When he has cleared anger and pain away with the power feather, he announces your new Indian name. It is Light As a Feather. And that's exactly how you feel. Being relieved of the mental and emotional weight of anger and pain has relieved your body of weight. You no longer need fat to hold anger or to insulate against pain. You feel slim and trim inside and out.

The medicine man makes one last gesture. He hands you the power feather, giving you the power to heal yourself of anger and pain. Next time a stressful situation arises, use the true power of the feather to resolve it, and you won't need to resort to the false and binding power of anger.

As you hold the power feather in your hand, a playful breeze comes to visit, and because you're so light it lifts you right off the ground. Up to the treetops you float, and over the waterfall, feeling giddy and silly and happy in the arms of the wind. The breeze sets you down in whatever place you want to be. You're free!

When you tell your subconscious that you want to be free of the heaviness of anger and pain, it will bring to you the insights, people, and situations that will help free you. Engender this feeling of lightness within you whenever possible. When you think light as a feather, and feel light as a feather, you'll be Light As a Feather.

Fat Free

Think of your fat cells as prisoners locked up in the prison of your body. They're serving time in different cell blocks of your body—arms, stomach, hips, buttocks, thighs—because they've committed crimes and misdemeanors against your health and happiness.

Some fat cells are serving short sentences of only a few days. Their offenses are relatively mild: perhaps putting butter on the toast at breakfast, or not being able to resist eating that chicken skin. Other fat cells are in for months, even years, having committed serious crimes involving pounds of chocolate truffles, gallons of ice cream, dozens of double cheeseburgers, bags of potato chips, or mountains of cookies.

And then there are the repeat offenders. These fat cells are released, and then a day, or a week, or a month later, they commit the same crimes and are right back in the slammer. Sometimes they come back bigger and badder than ever. The repeat offenders could end up serving life sentences if something isn't done.

As the warden of your fat prison, you're in charge of the fat cells, but trying to control your prisoners takes an enormous amount of time and energy. It's exhausting, debilitating, and frustrating. You *could* be using that time and energy to have fun and be healthy.

Do you really want to be the warden of a fat prison the rest of your life? How about using your position of authority to help rehabilitate the prisoners so they can be set free?

The first step in rehabilitating your fat prisoners is to tour the different cell blocks and observe the prisoners. Maybe you go to the stomach cell block first. What does it look like? What shape is it? What shape is it in? Is it bright and well maintained, or sagging and dingy? Are the prisoners crowded?

What do the stomach fat-cell prisoners look like? Fat, and sallow, and sad? What shape are they? What shape are they in? Are they human or cartoon-like? Are they male, female, or neuter? They could be round and firm, or soft and blobby. They might look like doughnuts with legs, or M&M's, or Jabba the Hut. Are they wearing prison uniforms?

What are the fat cells eating? Pizza and chocolate éclairs? What are they doing? They're probably just hanging around, bantering with each other and trying to impress each other with their size.

Hey, Slick, how ya hangin'?

•

You know what they say, "A pizza a day keeps everyone away."

•

So, Girth, it looks like you've been around.

What a waist!

Maybe you go to the buttock cell block next. What do these fat cells look like? What shape are they? What shape are they in? What are they eating? Milkshakes and doughnuts? What are they doing? Just sitting around?

Hey, Fat Cheeks, I see you've been sitting down on the job again.

•

How's that hindsight?

•

So, Mr. Bigshot, get a load of this.

The fat cells in different areas might look different. The thigh fat cells might be taller than the stomach cells, because they stand around. And from doing all that reaching, the upper arm cells might be thin compared to the hip cells, which are basically just along for the ride. Or you might picture all the fat cell prisoners looking the same.

Some prisoners are shackled by fear. Others are handcuffed by anger, or scarred with shame. All are imprisoned by pain. Being imprisoned in fat actually makes them feel safe.

After you've toured the prison and surveyed the activity—or lack of activity—of the fat cells, decide on the changes you want to make. How healthy do you want to be? How happy do you want to be? By how much do you want to reduce the fat prison population? Ten percent? Twenty-five percent? Fifty percent? Eighty percent?

Once you've decided on the changes you want to make—make them! Serve the fat prisoners healthy, nutritious food. See them eating fish, and salads, and fruits, and vegetables.

Picture the fat cells doing some form of exercise every day. It might be calisthenics, racquetball, jogging, basketball, swimming, bicycling, or walking.

Call in a wise and caring doctor to heal the fat cells of both physical and emotional maladies. What does the doctor look like? Man or woman? Young or old? What is he or she wearing? The doctor gives the fat cells shots of light and loving touches. He or she heals their fear, anger, shame, and pain with hugs and tender care. Compassionately, the doctor helps the fat cells understand that overeating was their solution to life's problems, pains, and pressures. He or she talks to the cell blocks of fat about alternative ways of coping: expressing emotions, asking for help, and being healthy.

The fat cells gain insight and lose guilt. They realize that they were coping in the only way they knew how, and are able to forgive themselves their food crimes. When they forgive themselves for being fat, a great weight is released.

See healing taking place. Maybe cells, or cell blocks, that were dark become light. Or areas that were tense relax. Or what was sour becomes sweet. Or what was loud becomes quiet. Or what was restless becomes calm.

As the prisoners regain their physical and emotional health, their entire demeanor improves. See or sense the fat cells slimming down. See their color brighten because they're in the pink of health. Feel how much they like being healthy.

Now that the fat cells are bright and healthy, prison has become confining. They feel crowded and frustrated by their lack of freedom. The fat cells want out. From every block of cells—arms, stomach, hips, buttocks, thighs—hear them chant in unison, "Free the fat! Free the fat! Free the fat!"

The doctor helps the fat cells plan for their release. They decide where they want to go when they leave. Some might want to go to the mountains, some to the seashore, some to favorite cities, or to fat farms. The prisoners are ready to be freed; they're at peace with the past and excited about the future.

You go before the judge and petition for the release of the prisoners. You point to the reformed fat cells, saying, "Judge, many of the cells you see before you have dealt with serious problems. Some were unloved or abandoned as children and ate to fill the emptiness. Some were abused—emotionally, physically, or sexually—and ate to ease the pain. Some were frightened and ate to barricade themselves against fear. Some were under tremendous pressure and ate to relieve stress. But they've learned how to cope with problems, pain, and pressure in constructive ways. They're healthy. Set them free!"

The doctor testifies to the emotional and physical health of the prisoners. People who love you and want you to be healthy are seated in the court and applaud your petition.

The judge is impressed with the changes you've made. He or she bangs the gavel and announces, "The prisoners are free to go." The people who love you cheer and whistle.

A chorus of fat cells sing good-bye and thank you for setting them free. They also sing to the doctor, thanking him or her for healing them. You're elated to see the fat cells looking so healthy, and acting so happy. Love and gladness grow within you, then burst out in bouquets of flowers. Flowers float out over all the used-to-want-to-be-fat cells.

Press the button that opens all the cell doors and the main gates in all the cell blocks. Where are the cell block gates located? In the stomach cell block the main gate might be in your belly button. In the thighs, the gates could be in your knees.

Fat cells begin pouring out of your body and into buses parked at every cell block gate. Knees, elbows, belly button, hips. What color and design are the buses? The buses have numbers that add up to the total number of pounds you want to release. The more weight you want to lose, the more buses there are, but if you want to lose ten pounds, there might be just one bus that stops at all the gates in your body. If you want to lose fifty pounds, there'll be a bus for each gate.

Picture the cells streaming into the buses. Hear them chanting, "We're free! We're free! We're free!" Each cell holds a flower.

Fat empties out of your body and into the waiting buses. As the buses fill up, they drive off. Who's driving the buses? The buses take off in all directions, transporting the fat cells away from your body to the destinations they've chosen.

Picture light and love filling the cell blocks where the fat cells were imprisoned. Filling the spaces with light will help prevent you from feeling empty and wishing that the fat cells were back again. What color is the light? What color is love? When you have replaced the fat cells with healthy, nonfattening lovelight, dance a little fat-free celebration jig.

In freeing the fat, you set yourself free. No longer a warden, you're free to use your time and energy to pursue whatever fulfills you. Your body is no longer a prison, but has been transformed into a home where your spirit, mind, and heart can grow in health and happiness.

This is a good visualization to do at the beginning of a diet. It can also be done periodically to free repeat offenders.

Snack Attackers

You've come to the conclusion that carrying around that extra poundage isn't providing pleasure, and you've decided to make a change for the better. Look out! As soon as you decide that some aspect of yourself needs changing, the very thing you want to change seems to take on a life of its own—a life it's willing to fight for. It's perfectly happy the way it is, thank you very much, and it's determined to maintain the status quo. In short, the thing you want to change, doesn't.

When you decide to make a change by losing weight, and begin backing up your thoughts with physical action, the habit of eating fattening foods resists. It digs in. It stands its ground. The more you try to change, the bigger and stronger the habit seems to become.

For example, you have a choice between eating an apple and eating a cupcake, and because you've decided to change the way you eat, you decide that eating the apple is the healthy choice. You reach for the apple, but an overwhelming urge for a cupcake takes over. The cupcake dances alluringly in your mind, large and in color. It sings sweetly to you in siren-like beseechments. You can smell it. You can feel it. You can taste it. Ya gotta have it.

Meanwhile the apple just sits there in the fruit bowl, or on the shelf in your refrigerator, minding its own business. It's being its sweet, crispy self, content in its healthfulness, with no need to exert control over you. You might make the smart move to eat it, or you might not; it's up to you.

The cupcake and the apple represent the warring sides of yourself. The cupcake represents the part of you that doesn't want you to be healthy and happy. It wants you to be fat, weak, unloved, or unsuccessful, or all the above. It doesn't want you to have the power to act positively on your behalf.

The apple represents the part of you that wants you to be healthy and happy. It wants you to be slim, fit, strong, loved, and successful. It wants you to be the best that you can be. It wants you to enjoy the power of taking action based on self-esteem.

If the unhealthy part of you isn't accurately symbolized by a cupcake, then picture the food that is most tempting: a cheeseburger, cookies, potato chips, or double chocolate fudge ice cream. Maybe the healthy part of you would be better represented by a salad, or pasta, or poached salmon. Visualize the foods that have the strongest appeal.

No matter what unhealthy fattening food lures you into its clutches, if you eat it, you'll give your power away to it. That means that you allow a cupcake to gain control of your mind and your body.

Come on. Seriously. Is a cupcake really stronger than you? Smarter than you? You're a living, thinking, feeling, human being; don't you have more on the ball than a Twinkie? Don't you think you can outsmart a cheeseburger?

Of course you can! On your worst day you're stronger and smarter than ground meat. Food only seems to control you because you let it. Food doesn't have power on its own; *you* give food power. You're the one making it big, strong, and attractive. The price you pay is that you make yourself big, weak, and unattractive. Selling your mind and body for a cupcake is a heavy price to pay, and you end up bankrupting your health and self-respect.

Use the power of your mind to strengthen the healthy part of you and be in control of what you eat. When alluring visions of cupcakes dance in your head, freeze-frame the image by thinking, *Stop!* Imagine yourself holding up a red and white hexagonal STOP sign in front of the dancing food. Maybe there's a Do Not Enter sign in front of your mouth.

If you feel that you need reinforcements, whistle for the Snack Attackers. They might be dogs who bark and growl menacingly at the cupcake, maybe sending it up a tree. Or the Snack Attackers could be a squad of your favorite linebackers, or cartoon characters, or food police. They form a barricade between you and temptation, and they can also pulverize unhealthy food with their laser guns.

At the same time as the Snack Attackers are providing extra muscle, you say to the food, mentally or aloud, "I am stronger than you!" Say it three times, each time louder and more forcefully. "I am stronger than you!" "I am stronger than you." The cupcake backs off.

Then say to the cupcake, "You no longer have the power to control me!" The cupcake moves farther away. Shout, "I refuse to allow you to control me!" The force of your words knocks the cupcake over. Yell, "You do not control me!" The cupcake begins to crumble.

Take your power back from the cupcake. Say, "Return my power to me. I demand that you give me back my power." See or sense power leaving the cupcake and taking some symbolic form in front of you. It might be an elixir of power that pours into a goblet for you to drink. It might be a seed of power. It might be a bowl of rainbows, or a plate of love. As the power that you had given to the cupcake leaves, the cupcake becomes smaller and smaller. It crumbles into a tiny pile.

Say "I reclaim my power!" As you say the words, reach out and take the goblet, or seed, or bowl, or plate of power in your mental hand, then eat or drink the contents.

Feel power sliding across your tongue and down your throat. What does it taste like? Sweet? Tart? What does it feel like? Effervescent? Silky? Cool? Warm? Power flows into your stomach, filling it. You feel satisfyingly full. Power is absorbed into your body, filling all the empty places. Every cell is nourished, becoming healthy and strong.

With the return of your power you feel whole and complete. You feel empowered and strong. Taking a long, deep breath, you exhale easily, blowing the remaining crumbs into oblivion. The healthy part of you is in charge. You radiate power, in control of your mind and your body.

Reach for the apple the same way you reached for your power. Eat it, noticing its sweet, crisp flavor; its texture and temperature. Let it fill your stomach in a satisfying way. Feel healthy nourishment being absorbed by your body.

Whenever unhealthy, fattening, power-draining food tries to control you, take action! Freeze-frame the image and take steps to regain your power. Be strong. Call in the Snack Attackers. The more you eat healthy food the stronger you become, and the easier it is to defeat the enticements of unhealthy food. When you think healthy, you'll eat healthy and be healthy.

Body Sculpting

Imagine that you're floating on your back in water. It might be a large pond or a lake. Or you can float in a saltwater sea, especially if you want extra buoyancy. Even if you're not good at floating in your physical reality, you're great at it in your mental reality. What color is the water? Aquamarine? Jade green?

Trust the water to completely support your weight. Your arms float out from your sides and your legs drift a comfortable distance apart. Your head rests on a pillow of water. What temperature is the water? Refreshingly cool? Soothingly warm? As you float on the water, you relax. Tension melts away.

Lying on your back, you look up at the blue sky arcing serenely above you. Sunlight slides through the air to touch your skin. Birds wheel overhead, celebrating this fine day with their calls. A breeze glides smoothly across the water. A friendly dolphin comes to visit, swimming around you once or twice in lazy circles, then leaping jubilantly into the air, splashing you gently with drops of sun-sparked water.

As you're floating on the water, feeling relaxed and happy, protected by the presence of the dolphin, you hear the sound of oars grinding in their oarlocks as paddles pull through the water. Let your legs drop down, and tread water to get a look at who's there.

The bow of a brightly painted rowboat is heading in your direction. What color is the rowboat? On the bow are the words *Ideal Form*. The boat skims across the water, drawing nearer and nearer.

Sitting in the rowboat are a man and a woman, each pulling an oar. What do they look like? They could be people you love who are living, or people you love who have died. They might be positive, powerful characters from a book, or a movie, or a cartoon. They could be people you don't know, whose images just pop into your mind.

Get as clear a sense of these two as you can. Notice the clothes they're wearing. The color of their hair. The color of their skin. The color of their eyes. The closer they row, the more details you can see. Regardless of their ages, they're both in great shape—ideal shape, in fact— and exude health and vitality.

When the boat is about fifteen feet away they hold the oars still to brake the boat, then hand the rope in the bow to the dolphin, who grasps it firmly in his beak, willingly serving as an anchor. The man and the woman turn to face you and say hello, calling you by name.

You return the greeting and, full of curiosity, ask, "Who are you? What are you doing here?"

The man and the woman smile merrily and lift their hands, flexing their fingers as if they were going to play a duet on a piano. "We're body sculptors. We're here to help form your ideal form." As the rower says "ideal form," he or she points to the side of the bow where the words are painted.

You laugh delightedly, saying, "Oh, I get it. Okay, let's do it!"

As soon as they know that you're agreeable to receiving their talented help, they stand up and shrug out of whatever they're wearing to reveal bathing suits. What design are they? Old-fashioned, modern, or futuristic? What color are the bathing suits? Out of what material are they made?

The man and the woman body sculptors dive off the side of the rowboat, slipping into the water with nary a ripple. The woman swims over to your left side, and the man swims around to your right side. They ask you to please float again. You do so, and in no time at all, you're as relaxed as you were before.

Again, the two lift their hands and flex their fingers. They ask you where you want them to begin to sculpt your ideal form. You tell them. Perhaps they start with your waist. Their hands feel warm and sure as they touch you, one on each side, gently massaging your waist. Using the tips of their fingers, they make small, gentle pulling motions around your waist downwards toward your feet, as if they were trying to catch the edge of a sheet of pastry dough that's been rolled out and is stuck on a board. But in this case it's your fat—including all the flour and butter you've consumed—that's stuck to your body.

They catch the edge of the fat that's settled around your waist, and begin to roll it down over your stomach, as you might roll down a wetsuit or a leotard. It doesn't hurt at all, and in fact, it feels rather pleasant. Once the fat starts rolling, the sculptors use their strong, deft hands to work it down your body. The fat rolls away from your waist, your stomach, and your hips.

Because you're suspended in water, the sculptors can get to every part of your body, front and back, at the same time. As they roll the fat over your abdomen, it also rolls away from your buttocks. The roll of fat becomes bigger and thicker. With each sculptor taking a leg, they roll the fat down your thighs to your knees, then down to your ankles. With a final tug they pull it off your feet. The sculptors are now holding your fat in their hands like a ball. Does it look like pastry dough? Or maybe clay? What color is it? How big is the ball of fat?

Swiftly and easily they have freed your entire lower body of fat. You feel appreciably lighter. The two body sculptors take the fat they've rolled off you, and toss it into the rowboat. *Thwunk.*

Where else do you want them to roll away fat? Your upper arms? The woman takes your left arm and the man takes your right. Using the tips of their fingers they make small pulling motions around your upper arms near your shoulders. They catch the edges of the fat and roll it down your arms to your elbows, then to your wrists. With a final tug they pull the fat over your hands and off. Again they toss the fat into the rowboat. *Thwunk.*

Sense your body. It definitely feels lighter and thinner. Are there any areas that could use a bit more sculpting? If so, tell the sculptors where. They roll more fat down and off, each time tossing the clumps of fat into the rowboat. *Thwunk.*

Then the body sculptors use their warm, sure hands to shape your body the way that's best for you. Your body curves in where it's supposed to, and out where it needs to. Your body feels firm and fit. You like the shape you're in. Being free of fat makes you feel more alive. This is your ideal form, and you love how it feels.

With heartfelt sincerity you thank the body sculptors for helping form your ideal form. They smile as they climb back into the rowboat and put their clothes back on.

The two body sculptors gather the fat they threw into the rowboat into one big ball. Out of the ball of fat they sculpt a statue of you when you were fat, capturing your likeness. The size of the statue reflects how much weight you want to lose. If your ideal form is many, many pounds less than you weigh now, the fat statue of you being fat will be almost as tall as you are, with proportioned torso and limbs. If reaching your ideal form means losing just a few pounds, then the statue will be in miniature.

The body sculptors place the fat statue in the bow, facing away from you, and take their seats. The dolphin offers up the rope, and one of them takes it from his beak. The dolphin squeaks goodbye, and clicks its approval of what has happened. Each sculptor gives you a smile and a wave good-bye, and then they begin to row away, taking with them the statue of your fat self.

You watch the rowboat pulling away, and soon you can no longer hear the oars grinding in the oarlocks. The boat, the ideal form sculptors, and your fat self become smaller and smaller, until they finally disappear. The dolphin does a grand celebration leap into the air, showering you with diamond drops, then swims a couple of lazy circles around you as you float peacefully and oh-so-lightly in the water. You're not just in good form today—you're in ideal form!

You can help attain and maintain your ideal body form by simply picturing the sculptors, one on either side of you, rolling the fat down from your body. Try doing this visualization when you're actually swimming, or even in a bathtub, to enhance the feeling of floating. This is a good one to do every day when you're first beginning to lose weight, and then every week as your fat loss gets rolling. It will also help you relax.

Thin Wins

The constant anxiety of adhering to a diet often makes you want to eat more. Instead of losing weight you end up losing peace of mind, self-respect, and control. You gain frustration, tension, and pounds. Struggle also binds the weight to you even more. The tension created by struggle becomes like a glue that makes fat adhere to your body. Here's a way to end the struggle, dissolve the glue, and release those pounds.

Imagine dieting as a tug of war between your fat self and your thin self; the diet is the rope. What animal would best represent your fat self? See that animal pulling on one end of the rope. Like a contestant in an athletic event, the animal has numbers tied to its front and back. The number on the front represents your current weight. The number on the back is the size of the clothes you wear.

What animal best represents your thin self? See that animal pulling on the other end of the rope. The number on the front represents how many pounds you weigh at your ideal weight. The number on the back is the size of the clothes you wear at your ideal weight.

Notice the rope. What color is it? How thick? How rough or smooth? How strong? Where does this tug of war take place? In your kitchen? In a restaurant? At work? In a dungeon? On a beach? In the desert? Does it take place mostly during the day or at night?

Walk around your fat-self animal and your thin-self animal so you can see them from all angles. Notice details about them, the rope, and the environment. Make the colors vivid. Smell the air. Hear the sounds of struggle. Touch your two animal selves. What do they feel like? Touch the rope. Touch the ground or floor.

Midway between the two animals a line has been painted on the ground or the floor. Painted on the fat one's side of the line is the word *Gain*. Painted on the thin one's side is the word *Lose*.

Back and forth, to and fro, the two animals go. They lose and gain, lose and gain. Fat. Thin. Fat. Thin. Fat. Neither your thin self nor your fat self looks happy. Both grimace and grunt as they struggle for control. What do they say to each other? Words and sentences, maybe epithets, pop into your mind.

The fat animal, being bigger, can throw a lot of weight behind its efforts. The thin animal is exhausted, but digs in. With valiant effort the thin animal grips the rope with tightly clenched and blistered paws, or hands, or hooves. Its arms, shoulders, neck and back ache with the strain of the struggle. The thin animal falters and falls. With smug superiority the fat animal drags the thin animal over the line. The result is that you eat what you had resolved not to, and too much of it. You gain weight.

This is a typical diet scenario acted out several times each day. How can your thin self win? A frustrating, exhausting, and painful tug of war with your fat self isn't the answer.

There *is* a way your thin self can win. Picture the fat and the thin animals pulling on the rope as you first did. Walk around, seeing them from all angles. Notice how unhappy and tired they both look. Hear what they say to each other. As you're walking around, the solution flashes through your mind like a comet.

Thin wins by letting go of the rope. See the thin animal let go of the rope with a big smile. See the fat animal fall, a surprised expression on its face as its rump hits the ground with a thud. It has nothing more than a bunch of slack rope to show for its efforts.

By not playing the diet game and not engaging in struggle, the smaller thin animal triumphs over the larger fat animal. By letting go of the rope, you let go of tension. When you let go of tension, the fat animal self falls because it was the tension on the rope that kept it upright. Once the fat animal falls, it's probably too fat to get up again. And even if it does manage to get up, as long as the thin animal refuses to engage in a diet tug of war, it can't play the game.

As soon as you see the thin animal drop the rope, and the fat animal falls with a thud, you feel an immense relief blow through your mind and your body. When you drop the rope, you free yourself from the struggle of dieting. You're free to be thin! You dance and leap for joy. Your hands, which were cramped and blistered from pulling on the rope, suddenly feel so light they could float in the air. Relieved of the rope, your hands are free to hold the things you want and the people you like, and bring them to you. The pain in your neck, and shoulders, and arms, and back disappears.

What a tremendous relief it is not to struggle with a diet. You think about how and what you're going to eat now that you're not on a diet. New possibilities open up. It occurs to you that combining thinking thin with the freedom of eating what you want can actually work in three ways. When you feed your subconscious mind happy, colorful pictures of you being happy and colorful at your ideal weight:

1. Your subconscious will make those pictures a reality by helping you *want* to eat healthy foods in healthy quantities.
2. By thinking thin, your body will digest food and burn fat more efficiently.
3. Even when you do want to eat pizza, or ice cream, or chocolate you'll satisfy the want in healthy moderation. You won't overeat as a result of the tension caused by struggle.

Your fat self and your thin self tried the diet tug of war and it didn't work. In dropping the diet you stop the struggle. You gain freedom, self-respect, self-control, confidence, and peace. Losing is gaining. Thin wins!

Not Stuck on You

Imagine that you're walking through a forest. Early-morning sun slants shyly through the leaves of the trees, dappling the leaf-and-moss-covered ground with soft light. Ahead, where the forest ends, the light widens and is bright. Your step, however, is heavy. Your feet are dragging as if the ground were covered with rubber cement instead of pine needles, making each step an effort. But you press forward.

Stepping out of the edge of the forest, you find yourself in an open meadow filled with sunlight and flowers. Bees drone low over lavender and white clover, and birds fly in high circles in the sky.

In the middle of the meadow is a large metal sphere made of iron. It's about eight feet in diameter. What color is it? Is it the color of iron, or has it been painted or electroplated? The sphere might be silver or gold, or cobalt blue, or have fuchsia polka dots. On the curved side facing you is a door. Is the door the same color as the rest of the sphere, or another color?

Drawn by your curiosity, you walk closer to the large metal ball resting in the middle of the meadow. A robin has perched atop its curved top and is singing its joy to the world, but within the ball itself, all is quiet. Not a peep.

Closer now, you can see the writing on the door:

I roll around,
Round and free,
Don't be stuck,
Be stuck on me.

Are the words printed or scripted? Are they etched or painted? What color are the letters?

Beside the door is a switch with a sign that reads, "Flip Me On." You do so, then curiously but cautiously open the door. It squeaks just a bit on its hinges, and hits the side of the metal sphere. *Thwank.* Inside, the convex walls are shiny and completely bare. What color is the inside of the metal ball?

Still standing on the doorsill, you see four steps leading down to the center of the curved floor. You walk down the steps to stand in the center, the shiny bright walls curving all around you. Looking down, you see a push-button switch and another sign:

Be a free and shining star,
Take your dreams out of the jar.
Then spread your arms to each side,
And spread your legs, not too wide.
Put your foot down.

Spread your arms out, your feet two feet apart, and put your foot down on the switch. First there's a whirring sound, and then a steady hum settles in. The metal ball becomes a powerful 360-degree magnet. It's ready to attract anything and everything within you and around you that you don't want. It does it easily and painlessly.

Tension pops out of your body and gets sucked to the sides of the ball. What color is the tension? What size? What consistency? What sound does it make as it hits the walls of the ball?

Anger follows suit. What color and consistency is it?

Aches and pains, both physical and emotional, are easily pulled out of you and adhere to the magnetized metal walls.

Layers of fat painlessly peel off your body and fly through the air to stick to the walls of the ball.

If unfriendly bacteria or viruses inhabit your body, sense/see them shooting out of your pores like bullets and spraying the walls.

Limiting or destructive thoughts are pulled from your head.

Thud. Thunk. Thwank. Squish. Plop. Bang. Rat-a-tat. Ping. Pang. Pong. Anything and everything you don't want in you, or on you, or around you, is painlessly pulled from you and immediately sucked to the powerfully magnetized walls.

You look around the curved walls at the clumps, and wads, and stains, and smears, and pits, and filings stuck there. All your unwanted negativity—tension, anger, pain, weight, worry, and disease—is held fast by the positive magnetic current. Not only is the current holding your negativity to the walls of the ball, but it is causing all that material to disintegrate. The bumps, and tufts, and knots, and globs of unwanted negativity are being cremated by the powerful positive current. It's all turning to ashes.

You feel abuzz with health. You glow with well-being. Positive energy flows through you. Walking up the four steps to the door, you notice that your step is markedly lighter and quicker.

Go out through the door. The sign by the switch now reads "Flip Me Off." You do so and the humming ceases. Everything that was stuck to the sides of the walls has now turned to ashes, and falls to the bottom of the sphere where you stood. A trap door opens and the ashes fall to the ground, where they will help to fertilize the earth.

Close the door. *Thwank.* You feel relieved of all kinds of weight, and are grateful that the sphere was there to help you. Humming a happy little tune, you look back at the sphere and see that it's rolling around, round and free. Sunlight and flowers spread around you. Your step is light, even jaunty, because you're not stuck, and nothing's stuck on you.

The sphere, with its powerful magnetic energy, will be there whenever you visualize it, to help free you of weighty concerns. This is a good visualization to do in the morning to help you move lightly through the day, and at night to free yourself of any weights you have acquired, so that you can rest easy.

Child Care

Overeating doesn't happen by itself. Something within you makes it happen. It's very likely that at least one of the events in your life that triggers overeating happened when you were a child.

There might have been an event that left you with an overwhelming sense of failure: anything from feeling responsible for your parents' divorce, to being the last one chosen for a team.

•

Maybe you were severely or constantly criticized by someone you looked up to, and made to feel worthless.

•

You may have suffered physical, mental, emotional, or sexual abuse.

•

You may not have been loved in the way you needed to be loved.

•

Someone may have humiliated you.

•

You may have been overprotected and so learned to fear life.

Your family might have been dysfunctional, unable to show you how to express emotions in a healthy way, or how to solve problems, so you were unable to learn healthy ways of coping.

Any of these events could have caused you to look for solace in food. At the moment that you're eating, food seems to fill the emptiness, insulate against pain, calm fears, and relieve stress. It temporarily distracts you from facing problems. Food doesn't criticize, frighten, abuse, or humiliate you. Eventually, of course, the food you've eaten too much of causes you to be fat, which can result in the same painful emotions you were using it to avoid.

When you overeat it could be partly because there's still a child within you who hurts, who even rages out of control, and uses the only thing he or she knows that helps: food. Because the past and the present are equally real to your subconscious, the feelings of your inner child are as alive now as they were many years ago. The wants and needs of your inner child can influence your adult eating behavior. Your inner child might be panicked with fear and starved for love, causing the adult you to eat for two. This visualization will help you find your child self and fill him or her with love.

Where do you think you'd be most likely to find your child self? In the house you lived in as a child? Or at a neighbor's house, at school, or at a store? In what room would your child self be, and what would he or she be doing? Playing, studying, watching television, reading, eating, sleeping, or hiding?

Find your child. (If the first image that comes to mind is of your child in a dangerous or unpleasant situation, bundle him or her right out of there to somewhere safe and peaceful, and continue the visualization from there.) About what age does she seem to be? What does your child look like? What is she wearing? How is she feeling? Are there smiles or tears?

When you locate your child, introduce yourself. Tell her your name as it is now. Ask your child her name. It might be the same first name as you have now, or a pet name you were called at that age, or a nickname. Whatever name pops into your mind—that's the one. Ask her how old she is.

Care for your inner child as you would like to have been cared for at that age. Tell her you'd like to be friends. How eager your child is for friendship will depend on how happy or sad she feels. If she's extremely agitated, hurt, or angry, she could be resistant to your overtures. Persevere. Ask if she'd like to go outside and play with you.

If your child sits there locked in pain or anger, put your arms around her saying, "You're feeling sad (or angry), aren't you?" She nods. Ask, "What can I do to help?" If she doesn't answer, ask, "Is there something you want?" Your child self nods again. "Tell me what it is," you say.

She could be suspicious of your offer, afraid of what you'll want in return. Reassure her, explaining that she doesn't have to do, say, eat, give, or be anything in particular to earn it. Tell your child that you want to give her something just because you love her. Say, "Tell me just one thing you want." Your child self tells you.

Your inner child could want anything from a horse to a hug: pets, games, playtime, clothes, jewelry, money, or food. Whatever it is, wrap it up, or tie a bow around it. Give your child the gift immediately and unconditionally, along with a hug.

Your child receives the gift with bright delight. She uses it, or does it, or wears it, smiling all the while. After receiving the gift, your child self feels calmer. Ask what else she wants, again giving it to her immediately and unconditionally, along with a hug. Give her a kitten, a puppy, a baseball mitt, a camera, a new sweater, a book, a bike, a video, a ring, a watch, even a birthday cake. Your child is filled with the understanding that she can receive what she wants without having to pay a price for it—she only has to be herself.

Compliment your child. Say something nice about a physical feature such as her hair or eyes. Tell her how smart she is, or athletic, or creative—or all three. Admire her talent, her spontaneity, the way she laughs, her loyalty, or how energetic she is. Tell your child every good thing about her. Fill her up with compliments.

Does your child like the clothes she has on? If not, let her pick out what she wants to wear. Ask if there's something she'd like to do. Let her do it, and even join in. Ask if there's somewhere special she'd like to go. Put her in a red wagon, or on a magic carpet, and take her there at the speed of thought. Maybe you go to Disney

World, or have a picnic at the beach, or hike through the mountains, or go shopping, or out to eat.

Find out what your child self wants and needs, and give it to her with no strings attached. Play with her and laugh with her. Get to know her by talking *with* her. Tell her that you want to be her friend. Listen to how she feels, and share with her how you feel.

Make her environment safe for her. As the adult, intervene between her and any abusers, protecting her. If your child doesn't feel safe where she is, take her somewhere where she will. Hold her and comfort her.

Every conversation, every gift, every trip, and every hug lets your child self know that he or she is loved. When you're first getting to know your inner child, try to spend at least a couple of minutes a day talking and playing with her.

Be the parent or friend your child didn't have. The more you know one another, the more trust develops, and the more love grows. When your inner child feels full of love, he or she won't need food to fill the emptiness, and you can eat just for one. Take care of yourself by caring for the child within.

Well Suited

You're getting dressed to go to work or out for the evening, but none of the clothes in your closet seem to suit you. You don't like the color. Or you don't like the design. Or you don't like the fit. Or the fit doesn't like you. Or all of the above. You lift out one hanger of clothing after another, look at each one, and discard them in disgust.

Just when you're feeling so frustrated that you're considering not going out—maybe ever again—you notice a large oblong box in the back of the closet. The box might be propped against the wall, or lying on the shelf. It's wrapped like a gift and tied with a bow. What color is the wrapping paper? How big is the bow?

Curious as to what this present is doing in your closet, you pick it up. It isn't heavy, but when you shake it, something inside shifts. Tucked under the bow is a gift card, which you slide out and open. It reads To (your name), From (your name) With Love, To Help You Think Thin and BE Thin! It's a gift from you to you, from the part of you that loves yourself and wants you to be healthy and happy, to the part of you that doesn't.

Reading the card makes you even more curious. Eagerly you slide off the ribbon and tear off the wrapping paper. Excitedly you lift off the lid of the box and push aside the brightly colored tissue paper. Nestled in the paper is a soft, thick, terry cloth jump suit with a zipper up the front. You lift it out and look at it. It has feet like the pajamas little children wear, and mittens for your hands. It also has a close fitting hood.

What color is the jump suit? Does it have designs on it? Is it striped, or plaid, or plain? Maybe your initials are embroidered on it. Or stars. Maybe there's a large red heart on the front. The words *Think Thin* could be printed all over the jump suit in gaily colored letters, or just on the key areas that you want to be thinner. Picture the jump suit so that it suits you.

Check the label in the neck band for the size. It might be sized by letter: XL, L, M. Or by number: 20, 16, 14, 12, 10. Discovering that it's just your size, you read the care instructions:

This material contains fat-absorbent Thinalin.
Non-irritating. Wear daily.
Wash, dry clean, or incinerate. No ironing needed.

It dawns on you that the jump suit is going to help absorb fat from your body. You're so excited that you can hardly wait to put it on. You take off the clothes you're wearing, and with glee unzip the zipper. Is the zipper gold or silver? Jump into the jump suit. Your feet fit perfectly in the jump suit feet. Pull it up past your waist and push your hands through the armholes, down the sleeves into the mittens, then shrug it up over your shoulders. Pull the hood up over the back of your head, feeling it fit snugly over your ears. The jump suit fits like a glove. The soft, fluffy terry cloth feels soothing against your skin.

With a flourish you pull up the zipper. Hear the sound it makes as it closes the jump suit from your navel to your neck. Pulling up the zipper activates the *Thinalin*, which immediately begins absorbing fat from your body with a gentle wicking action like a towel absorbing water. The sensation is that of a gentle pulling, or a slight tingling. The process is as painless as drying yourself after a bath or shower.

You can tell that the *Thinalin* is working because stains begin appearing on the jump suit over the areas of fat: stomach, hips, thighs, waist, arms, and so on. The stains might be a darker shade of whatever color the jump suit is, or they might turn brown, gray, or even black, depending on how much fat there is to absorb. The close fitting hood turns dark as it pulls fat thoughts from your mind.

You might also notice dark stains appearing on the jump suit over areas that aren't really fat, like an elbow. This is because the terry cloth jump suit, in addition to soaking up fat from your body, also absorbs tension, disease, injury, toxins, and pain—both physical and emotional. A stain over your heart area might be fat, or it might represent emotional pain.

Whatever weighs you down, whether physical or emotional, can be released into the jump suit. Allow this release to happen. Encourage it. Verbally give your body permission to release fat and pain. Say: "I give every cell in my body permission to let go of unnecessary fat." Then say, "I give every cell in my body permission to be free of pain."

As the jump suit wicks away fat and pain from your body, and you see different areas of the jump suit turn dark, you feel decidedly lighter. Not only does your body feel less weighed down, but so does your mind. Your attitude brightens. You feel less encumbered both physically and emotionally.

When the wicking action seems to have stopped, unzip the jump suit, peel back the hood, shrug your arms out of the sleeves, push the jump suit down to your feet, and step out of it. The terry cloth that was soft and fluffy will now feel stiff and hard with the fat and toxins it has absorbed.

After you take off the jump suit, check yourself out in a full-length mirror. See a thinner, trimmer you reflected there. Your skin has a healthy glow. Your hair shines. Your eyes sparkle. You like what you see and a big smile spreads across your face.

Picking up the clothes you were wearing before you put on the jump suit, you put them on, but they're big on you now and hang unattractively. Quickly you take them off again and hunt through your closet for something to wear that suits the new you. To the right, in the back, hanging on a hanger with a balloon tied to the hoop, are clothes that you hadn't noticed before. They're exactly the style, color, and fit that are most becoming to you. Eagerly you put them on, and check yourself out in the mirror again. Yes. This suits you perfectly.

The stained, crusty jump suit lies crumpled on the floor. You pick it up between two fingers, holding it away from you, and toss it in the washing machine. Or take it to the cleaners. Or throw it in a roaring fire, hearing the fat crackle as it burns.

However you clean your jump suit, it comes out fresh and fluffy, without a stain on it, but it doesn't lose any *Thinalin*. If you prefer to simply dispose of the jump suit, there'll always be another one waiting for you when you want it. Check the label in the neck from time to time, and you'll see the size change as your size changes. As you shrink, the jump suit will shrink.

It helps to wear your fat-absorbing jump suit twice a day. Put it on in the morning while you're brushing your teeth, or shaving, or putting on your make-up, to help you start the day off on the right track, the thin track. Slip into it again at night to help absorb any fat that might have accumulated during the day. Wearing it while you sleep will help those pounds melt away, and you may even have dreams of being thinner. Your *Thinalin* jump suit is well suited to helping you think thin and be thin.

Taming the Beast

Instead of that lovin' feelin', you've got that empty feelin'. A bad case of the "empties" is gnawing away inside you, weakening your willpower. You may not even actually feel physically hungry, just restless, nervous, or incomplete. The thought of something sweet and gooey—and lots of it to fill that empty space—is becoming more appealing with each passing beat of your heart. And just when you've been so good about your diet.

Quick! Before you completely lose your resolve, get a grip! Get control. Fill up the emptiness.

First, get a fix on just where the emptiness is located. Is it in your stomach? High or low? Left or right of center? Lower abdomen? Lower back? Is it in your solar plexus? Or is it your heart that feels empty?

That empty feeling could be anywhere in your body, so keep an open mind about its location. Don't cancel out the information your subconscious gives you with conscious mind judgments, because even your elbow or your ear can feel empty.

Once you've located the empty feeling, give form to the emptiness so you can get a handle on it. If the emptiness were an animal, what kind of animal would it be? Do you see it as a buck-toothed beaver gnawing away? A hungry, roaring lion? A squealing pig caught in a barbed-wire fence of anger? A horse galloping away across the plains of your emotions, wild and out of control? A long-tailed rat scurrying hither and thither looking for something on which to chew? A bird fluttering helplessly against the bars of a cage? A cat—kitty or tiger—with claws extended, scratching for food and attention?

If the emptiness animal makes you nervous, or frightens you in any way, create something to protect yourself. You might visualize a fence or a plastic shield around yourself, or around it. Control the animal with your voice, or keep it at bay by cracking your whip.

Once you feel confident that your emptiness animal can't hurt you, form a clear picture, or sense, of it. Use your mind and your heart to know how it looks and moves and what sound it makes. Is its scent pleasant or unpleasant? If you feel comfortable doing so, reach out a hand and touch it. What does it feel like? How warm or cool is it?

Talk to your emptiness. Does it have a name? Tell it how you feel about it. Are you scared of it? Does it make you feel helpless? Does it confuse you? Does it make you feel sad? Does it annoy you? Or is it your only friend?

Ask the emptiness animal how it feels about you. Does it like you, or is it frightened of you? Is it angry with you?

Is there something that it wants from you that you haven't been giving it? Find out by asking, "What do you want? What do you need?" It might want to play with you. Or take you somewhere to show you something. Maybe it wants you to pet it. It might need understanding or forgiveness. It might be hungry for something either literal or symbolic. The animal might say it wants a bowl of ice cream, or attention and love. Whatever it wants, provide it. With your mind's eye, picture the thing your emptiness animal wants, and give it plenty of it. When the hunger animal is full, it will stop gnawing at your insides and go away. When the animal leaves, so does the emptiness.

Whenever you've got that empty feelin', locate its place in your body, and then picture or sense it as an animal. It might be the same animal each time you do the visualization, or it might be a different one. Then take charge and feed it so it goes away. When you rid yourself of emptiness in your mind, you help rid yourself of emptiness in your body.

Restaurant of Your Dreams

In order to get what you want, it helps to know what you want. If you don't, the results are the same as going into a restaurant and not being able to tell the waiter what you want. Either you'll get nothing and be hungry, which will make you cranky and cause you to overeat when you get home, or you'll get food you don't like, which will also make you grumpy, and you'll still overeat when you get home.

The solution to this sorry scenario is to know what you want and ask for it. Picture yourself going to eat at the Restaurant of Your Dreams. What does the entrance look like? Walk in the door. The maitre d' seats you at a plush banquette and hands you a menu. He unfolds the napkin in front of you, and you see that it's the lace napkin from your Palace of Power, monogrammed with your initials. With a flourish, the waiter places the napkin on your lap.

Open the menu and find all your needs and desires listed. Some, such as wanting a new calculator, or parking spaces, or to wake up happy, are appetizers. Others— wanting a new car, a better job, a thinner body, the answer to a problem, a lovemate—are main courses. Still others are desserts, such as receiving a present or having sweet dreams.

As you're looking at your dream menu, your Pal from the Palace of Power slides in across the table from you. A waiter brings his special napkin, embroidered with his name and an ace of hearts. As you greet each other you realize that the Restaurant of Your Dreams is in your Palace of Power. Your Palace Pal says, "Don't forget, the waiter is here to bring you *anything you want,* but you have to ask for it." Right, but what *do* you want? Look at your menu of wants and pick one. Give your order to the waiter, who writes it down, then punches it into a computer where it's instantly displayed in the kitchen for the chef to prepare.

Say you order a thinner body. If the waiter emerges from the kitchen with a body that's the same shape as the one you have now, or even fatter, it means that your order got scrambled. Either you didn't state what you wanted clearly, or some contrary belief contradicted it.

Send the fat body back. Then, to prevent the order from getting bollixed up again, go downstairs to the *Basement of Beliefs.* When you open the door marked *Beliefs,* you find a room with a table, a throne, a file cabinet, and a fireplace. A fire is burning in the fireplace, and lying on the table are a black marker and a gold pen. What other furnishings are in the room?

Pulling open a drawer in the file cabinet, you find a thick ledger with alphabetic index tabs. The ledger contains your beliefs about every aspect of your life: beliefs that either help or hinder your success. Bring the ledger over to the table, pull up your throne, and sit down. Open the ledger to the *w*'s for *Weight.*

On the page you open to is written, in your hand-writing, the following belief: "Losing weight is difficult." Pick up the black marking pen and write *Void* or *No* across the page in big letters. Then tear out the page and tear it into pieces. Throw the pieces into the fire. The negative belief, with its power to interfere with positive goals, turns to ash.

Open the ledger to a fresh page, pick up the gold pen, and write a new belief: "Losing weight is easy." See the words written in gold, in your handwriting. Touch the words with your hand. The power of the words leaps into your hand, up your arm, through your neck, and into your mind. Imbued with the strength of the belief that losing weight is easy, you'll lose weight more easily.

Go back upstairs to the dining room in the Restaurant of Your Dreams, and place your order again. Give the waiter a clear description of the thinner body you want by drawing him a mental picture of it. The waiter clicks his heels together as soon as he receives the order, and this time he personally takes your order to the chef.

With no negative belief about losing weight to countermand your order, you should get what you want. The waiter emerges from the dream kitchen pushing a large cart in front of him. On the cart is your thinner body, just the way you ordered it. The waiter places it on your lap. What does your thinner body feel like sitting on your lap? Lighter? Firmer?

You love your thinner body so much that you give it a big hug. As soon as you hug your thinner body, it merges with you. Pop! You become thinner. Getting what you ordered makes you one happy person. You feel full. The waiter and your Pal applaud your ordering mastery. The restaurant bells peal in celebration. Three cheers. *Clap, clap, clap. Peal, peal, peal.*

This is an especially fun and helpful visualization to do when you actually go to a restaurant. As you're perusing the menu, be thinking about the thinner body you want. When you order, you'll get what you want.

Light Snack

Instead of ordering an ice cream shake to fill an empty stomach, order up a light shake—it's packed with energy and has zero calories. Picture, or sense, yourself pouring thick, creamy liquid light into a large metal shaker. What flavor light do you have a taste for? If it's a vanilla shake you want, you'll see the light as white, while yellow is for banana, pink for strawberry, blue for blueberry, and so on. You have all the colors and flavors of the rainbow from which to choose, so make it tasty.

Mix and match to your heart's content. You might want to add success protein powder, or a raw egg of golden energy, or diamond dust for fiber and sparkle. Use your imagination—and add that, too. Sweeten with honey-love and blend on high self-esteem.

When you've made your light shake just the way you want it, pour it into a glass. Feel the cool, smooth surface of the glass as your fingers close around it. Lift it to your mouth, and let the sweet, creamy light flow across your tongue, tickling your tastebuds. Take time to be aware of the taste of the light and the feel of it on your tongue.

Swallow, letting the rich liquid light slide down to your waiting stomach. Picture your stomach filling up with light. See the flavor color of the light shake you whipped up flowing into every nook and cranny of your stomach, until there is no empty space left.

Feel your stomach filling up. Feel the light pouring in and chasing away the emptiness. As you sense your stomach becoming comfortably full, you give your subconscious the message that you *are* full. The light coats your stomach, soothing it, and, whenever you eat, the light helps digest your food more efficiently. You might even experience a sensation of warmth or tingling in the area of your stomach as you assimilate light energy into your body.

Keep your stomach full of light all through the day, and all through the night. Picture rich, creamy light filling your stomach as soon as you wake up, and the last thing before you go to sleep. This is one meal that allows you to sleep on a full stomach. Light also makes a great in-between-meal snack. High in energy and low in fat, you'll fill up on light, but you won't fill out.

Round 'Em Up

Imagine that your fat cells are like sheep spread out over the hills and plains of your body. You're a rancher and have just made a deal to trade your fat, woolly sheep for lean, powerful horses. What do you need to do to efficiently and quickly move the sheep off your land and bring in the horses?

Herding all those sheep on foot would be difficult and time-consuming, so do it on horseback. As soon as you think *horseback*, you find yourself sitting astride a powerful stallion. What color is he? What name do you give him? The reins are firmly in your hands, and despite the horse's size and strength, it takes only the most gentle tug for the horse to respond to your commands.

Sitting high on your horse, atop a peak in Mind Mountain, you feel strong and capable. From that vantage point, survey your body. See the hills and valleys where flocks of fat woolly sheep graze.

How large are the flocks? Could you use some help in rounding them up? Picture people who love you and want to help on horseback next to you, dressed in cowperson outfits. They might be relatives, friends, coworkers, your doctor, and so on. Sitting on one horse is a surprise helper. It might be a shepherd from ancient times, or a Teenage Mutant Ninja Turtle, or your fairy godmother. And what would a sheep roundup be without sheep dogs? See several.

If you see people who want to prevent you from rounding up the sheep, throw a lasso around them, binding their arms, then jerk their legs out from under them and turn them over to the sheriff. The sheriff arrests them on charges of trespassing and obstruction of justice, and puts them in jail.

The air is crisp and filled with the barking of the sheep dogs and the whinnying of the horses. The horses paw the ground, eager to be on their way. Before setting out, check to see if there are any fat-sheep thoughts on Mind Mountain. If there are, round 'em up. Then shove your fist in the air and shout, "Ho!" You and your rounder-uppers ride off down the mountain and through Neck Gorge. The rounder-uppers agree to split into two groups to get any sheep that may have wandered into the canyons of your arms, leaving one person and a sheep dog to stay with the sheep from Mind Mountain.

Off you gallop with your group, the horses' hooves echoing on the rock surface of Shoulder Bluff, then down into narrow Arm Canyon West. Sheep might be caught in the rocks of the canyon walls, or they might be grazing down by the river. Wherever you spot sheep, ride around behind them shouting, "Git!" The other rounder-uppers do the same. The sheep are slow and not too bright, so they herd together obediently without giving you much trouble. The sheep dogs keep the sheep in line.

Herd your flock of fat sheep back up across Shoulder Bluff to join the sheep from Mind Mountain. The other group arrives with their flock of fat sheep from Arm Canyon East. The flock is getting larger. Are all the sheep the same color and size, or are sheep from different areas different colors? Move the entire flock down to Heart Cave. What does the Heart Cave look like? Check inside the cave for any lost sheep.

Leaving the Heart Cave, you, the rounder-uppers, and the sheep dogs move the flock down to a large holding pen in Great Stomach Bulge, where a big flock of sheep is already grazing. A few sheep try to break away from the flock, but the rounder-uppers and the dogs are too fast for them, and the sheep are brought back into the fat fold. What does the holding pen look like? How big is it?

Once all the sheep are penned in, everyone again decides to split into two groups. One group will take Hip Hill and Thigh Canyon West, and the other will round up sheep in Hip Hill and Thigh Canyon East. Leave a rounder-upper and a dog at Great Stomach Bulge to make sure that no sheep squeeze out of the pen.

You ride to Thigh Canyon first. As you ride, the powerful movements of the horse and the sound of his hooves pounding across the ground make you feel powerful. The roundup of fat sheep is going smoothly, and will soon be done. You feel proud of yourself for taking charge and maintaining control so easily. You're also grateful for all the help you've received.

Thigh Canyon is larger than Arm Canyon so there's a bit more territory to cover, but the sheep are docile and the roundup goes efficiently and quickly. How large is the flock? What size and color are the sheep? With the help of dogs, horses, and rounder-uppers, herd them over to Hip Hill, and round up however many fat sheep are grazing there. Then move the combined hip-and-thigh herd back to Stomach Bulge.

The holding pen expands automatically to hold the sheep you've brought in. It expands again when the second group brings in the sheep they have gathered. Look at the fat, woolly sheep crowded together in the pen. About how many are there? Hundreds? Thousands? If you think there might be sheep you've overlooked, ride out to those areas with your helpers, and bring them in.

As soon as you've gathered the fat sheep together from every part of your body, the person with whom you're doing the trade arrives in a spaceship. The spaceship is larger than the holding pen, and hovers over it. He's from the planet Waytoothin and his people need those fat, woolly sheep of yours. A column of red-white light the circumference of the holding pen descends from the spaceship to the ground, enfolding the sheep in light. Then the light retracts, lifting every single fat, woolly sheep into the cargo hold. Your weight is lifted, and your spirits lift.

As you and the rounder-uppers stand in stunned awe, another column of light descends. Again it's the circumference of the holding pen, but this time it's violet-white. In the violet-white light are held the most beautiful and handsome horses you have ever seen. The light lowers them gently to the ground, then snaps off. Every conceivable breed of horse is represented, from mottled Appaloosas to giant Clydesdales, their coats shining so, they almost glow.

You wave to the spaceship and it flashes its lights at you, then veers off into space, taking away your fat sheep. Your attention is drawn back to the magnificent horses. As soon as you look at them you realize that their energy and power shouldn't be held in. With a flick of your thought, make the holding pen disappear. The horses run free, spreading out in all directions, adding their energy to the hills and canyons of your body.

When the horses have galloped off you notice that the Great Stomach Bulge has disappeared. It was never a bulge at all; it was the fat, woolly sheep that made it bulge. Rename it Stomach Valley.

Your trusty horse stays with you, ever ready to take you around your body whenever you want, whether to survey the lay of the land, admire the horses, or look for stray sheep. Thank the rounder-uppers for their help, and pat the dogs. You don't need them now, but if you do, they'll be there.

Ride your horse back to your ranch house on Mind Mountain. Your body is no longer a sheep ranch crowded with slow, fat sheep: it's now a horse ranch where strong, fleet, powerful horses roam. When you need energy or power, get on your trusty horse and round 'em up!

Fat Vac

Does your body feel gritty from too much sugar? Grimy with starch? Gunked up with grease? Fubsy with fat? Suck it out and clean it up with Fat Vac, the all-purpose vacuum cleaner. You don't have one and don't know where to get one? You will by the end of this visualization.

Picture the door to the closet or cabinet where you keep your broom, mop, dustpan, and vacuum cleaner. Notice the appearance of the door, and put your fingers around the handle or knob that opens the door.

Opening the door, you see all your familiar cleaning implements. But look again; there's something in the closet that wasn't there before. It looks like an industrial-strength vacuum cleaner, and it says Fat Vac in big fat letters on the side of the canister.

Pull it out of the closet and take a good look at it. What color is the canister? If it's utilitarian gray or brown, change it to fun fuchsia, or lime green, or Day-Glo orange with lime green flocked polka dots. Is the hose the same color as the canister, or different, or striped? The suction nozzle is rounded like the one you use for upholstery. Is it metal or plastic?

Instructions are printed on the canister and you lean down to read them.

Vacuum all kinds of fat: fat fat, medium fat, slight fat. Plug in, turn on, apply nozzle to fat surfaces. Be sure to empty bag. Genii attachment optional.

Well, that sounds simple and straightforward enough. You check to see if you have the optional genii attachment. Yup. It says Genii Attachment, and it's hooked right onto the side of the canister. It looks ordinary, but you give it a little push to make sure it's firmly attached.

Pull or carry the vacuum cleaner into a room in your home where you feel especially relaxed and comfortable. What room is that? You might want to draw the curtains or blinds and close the door so you have total privacy.

Once the room is secure, turn your attention to the Fat Vac. Before plugging it in, make sure there's a new, empty fat bag. The electric cord might be wrapped around the vacuum, or it might be the kind you pull out from the back of the canister. Unwind it, or pull it out, and plug the plug into a convenient electrical outlet.

Turn on the switch. The Fat Vac hums to life and you grab the shaft of the nozzle. As you lift it up, you notice a cloud of mist emanating from the head of the nozzle. It blows out of the nozzle like steam and begins to take on the form of a genii, complete with turban, scimitar, and pointy brocade slippers.

It takes a moment for the genii to shape up, but when fully and firmly formed, he folds his arms across his bare chest and announces: "I am the fat Genii, Genii the Fat. The Lord of Thin, the Shah of Shape, the Sultan of Slim, the Prince of Poundage, the King of Fit. You can call me Genii, or you can call me Fat. Or you can call me Genii the Fat. Or you can call me Fred."

Greet the fat Genii by whichever name tickles your fancy, and introduce yourself. Genii the Fat bows to you, then, calling you by name, says, "You, (your name), have summoned me forth. Is it your wish to be less fat?"

You reply affirmatively. "Yes!"

The fat Genii says, "Your wish is granted." He takes the hose and nozzle from your hand, and brandishes it as he might his scimitar, with determination and vigor. But unlike using a scimitar, this separation of fat from body will be painless. It will be as swift and sure, but without pain. And the magic of the Fat Vac is that it only pulls out excess fat, leaving intact everything you need to be healthy.

Stand at ease in the center of the room, legs slightly apart, and arms hanging loosely by your sides. Genii the Fat puts the suction nozzle on your stomach, and moves it back and forth across the surface. The mild tugging action of the suction feels pleasant, even soothing. Your fat loses its hold on your body and is effortlessly sucked up through the hose and into the fat bag in the canister. What sound does the fat make as it's being sucked up through the hose?

The Genii moves the suction nozzle to every area of your body where you want to let go of fat. He moves the nozzle back and forth, pulling fat out of your body pain-lessly and effortlessly. Hear the sound the fat makes as it's sucked through the hose. Feel the fat leaving your body smoothly and easily. Feel it being sucked from your stomach, waist, hips, buttocks, and thighs. If you want to let go of fat in your arms, hold your arms out to let the fat Genii vacuum up the fat. If there are any areas Genii the Fat has missed, or that you want him to go over again, tell him where they are.

As the fat is suctioned up, out, and away, your body feels lighter and brighter. It feels clean, cleared of both physical and emotional heaviness. Your body feels increasingly lighter and tighter.

When all the fat that can be vacuumed by the Fat Vac has been sucked up, leaving the fat your body needs to maintain health, Genii the Fat puts down the hose and nozzle. He unplugs the Fat Vac and opens the canister to remove the now bulging fat bag. The fat's in the bag. Holding the bag in his left hand, the fat Genii faces you and folds his right arm across his bare chest. Looking you in the eye he winks and says, "You are less fat. Your wish has been granted. Summon me as needed."

You are truly happy to have your wish granted. You look down at your slimmer body. It looks great on the outside and feels great from the inside. Elated, you thank Genii the Fat for helping you become thin. He nods, then disappears in a puff of stuff, and the fat in the bag disappears with him.

Yes! You jump for the joy of being thinner, and because there's now less of you to elevate, you jump higher than you've ever jumped before. You're the Lord or Lady of Thin, the Prince or Princess of Poundage, the King or Queen of Fit.

Whenever you feel gritty, grimy, gunked up, or fubsy with fat, get out your Fat Vac. Check to make sure the genii attachment is attached, then plug it in, turn it on, and let the Genii of Fat vacuum excess fat out of your body.

Thin Is a State of Mind

Your thoughts affect your body. Positive thoughts have a positive effect on your body; negative thoughts have a negative effect. For instance, how you think about your body can affect how well it metabolizes food. Your thoughts about your body image will also affect your eating behavior, determining what you eat, how often you eat, and how much you eat. This cause-and-effect relationship makes your state of mind about your body an important consideration.

What's your state of mind about the size and shape of your body? Are you in a fat state of mind? Imagine that you're living in the state of Fat, and driving a big car that's a real gas guzzler. What color is the car? What model? What shape is it in? Does it often break down and require attention? Are you alone in the car, or is it packed with noisy people from your past and present who constantly criticize your driving?

The dirt road you're driving on makes you nervous because it's narrow and full of potholes. Much of the surrounding area looks as if it's been hit by a drought. What vegetation there was is now shriveled and brown. Several trees seem to have been hit by lightning, and their blackened remains are silhouetted against an overcast sky.

Homes along the way are cramped and crowded together. Inside, people are eating, watching television, and sleeping. On the streets people look bored and boring. They trudge along, bent over as if carrying large burdens, eyes glued to the ground. Stores are large, brightly lit, and well stocked, but they're all closed. The bank, too, has a Closed sign in its window.

If life looks physically, mentally, and emotionally impoverished to you, you could be in a depressed state. That's the bad news. The good news is that you don't have to live there. You're free to leave the state of Fat whenever you want, just as you can leave the geographical state you're living in if you decide to.

That's the key: deciding. What separates the state of Fat from the state of Thin is the line of decision. You decided to live in the state of Fat, and there you are. But wait, you protest, I didn't make any such decision; I was forced into it by my past, by people, by situations.

That kind of thinking is dangerous because it puts you in the role of a victim, with no power of your own. Without self-determination you're at the mercy of other people. You might not have consciously chosen to be in the state of Fat, but by not choosing to live in the state of Thin, you ended up in the state of Fat by default.

As you're driving along, kicking up a cloud of dust behind you, you see a shiny sign to your right. In bright letters on a clear background the sign announces STATE OF THIN—1 Block. What do you want to do? Stop? Turn around? Go ahead? What do you think? It's your decision.

Yes! Go for it! Put your foot down on the accelerator and head for Thin. As soon as you decide to go to Thin, the road widens, becomes paved, and the potholes disappear. Just making the decision fills you with glee.

As you approach the Thin state line, you see a huge, white square trash can. On the side, in big block letters, it says THROW BLOCKS HERE. At first you wonder what it means, then you remember the sign that said: STATE OF THIN—1 Block. What is the number one block you have against being thin? Look down at your lap and see a block there. How big is it? How heavy? Is it a wooden block or a cement block? On it is printed, also in block letters, No. 1, and the name of whatever it is that blocks you from being thin. The block might say *fear, pain, anger, self-disgust, jealousy, envy, hopelessness, victimhood, resentment, bitterness,* and so on.

Roll down the window and pull even with the garbage can. Heave whatever your block is to being thin into the can. Hear the sound it makes as it hits the inside of the can and falls to the bottom. Whew! What a relief to get rid of that block. If you have other blocks, throw them in the garbage, too.

As soon as you cross the line you see a sign that announces ENTERING THE STATE OF THIN. This is a pleasant, healthy state to be in. The road you're on is smooth and in good repair. It's paved with an all-weather surface and is four lanes wide. The surrounding area looks like an oasis. Flowers and fruit trees are everywhere, the air redolent with their sweet aromas.

Homes along the way are large, well maintained, and have big yards. Inside some of the homes people are eating together around a table, talking and laughing, and enjoying each other's company. In other homes people are reading, listening to music—or playing it—pursuing a hobby, or doing a little extra work because they like what they do.

On the streets people walk briskly, full of purpose and energy. They look fit and their eyes gleam with dreams for the future. The stores are large, brightly lit, and well stocked. Every store is open, and so is the bank.

The state of Thin looks so lively and interesting that you decide to stop and see it up close. Get out of your car and cross the street; the median is planted with flowers. Stop and smell the roses. You go into the bank, and the teller addresses you by name. Write a check for however much money you need; the teller cashes it and puts the money in your hand. Do a little shopping. The salespeople all know you by name, and gladly help you pick out what you want.

It pleases you deeply to have gained so many things you wanted and needed. A tall, friendly rabbit walking on the street helps carry your packages. You cross the street to where you parked your car, but the big old gas-guzzler you arrived in is gone. Bewildered, you look around. Panic starts to build. Where's your car? It was big, but it was yours. How are you going to get around? "If you please, very well," says the rabbit. You hadn't realized that you'd spoken aloud.

The helpful rabbit continues being helpful by explaining what happened to your car. "When you come to the state of Thin, you no longer need a big car—not that yours wasn't perfectly okay—so the state automatically gives you a smaller car. This is it." In the exact spot where you had parked your fat car, there now sits a car one or more sizes smaller. It's the car you've been wanting. What make and model is it? What color? You're ecstatic.

From the radio antenna hangs a tag with your name on it, reading From the State of Thin with Love. The door is unlocked and the keys are in the ignition. Thank the helpful rabbit for being so helpful. Put your purchases inside the car and get in. The seat supports you firmly yet comfortably. Turn the key in the ignition and hear the engine purr with power.

As soon as you put your hands around the steering wheel you know that this is the car for you. The steering wheel feels custom fitted, and you grip it with a light but sure touch. With a wave to the rabbit, you drive off. The smaller car handles just the way you had hoped it would. It's responsive to your slightest touch and hugs the road with ease, even around sharp curves. It's so fuel-efficient that you can cruise for hours before needing gas. You realize that this car is going to be a lot easier and cheaper to maintain, too.

Turn the radio on. An announcer says, "And for your listening pleasure we're going to play a medley of thin tunes: 'I've Got Thin On My Mind,' 'What Would I Do Without Thin,' and 'Let's Stay in Thin.'" You can easily hear the songs because nobody's in the back seat telling you how to drive. Besides, in your smaller car, there's no room for bigmouths.

You're in charge and you love it. Honk for thin. Honk for joy. Honk for health.

Whenever you think you're fat, change your state of mind by driving right into the state of Thin. When you change your mind, you change your body.

Fat Elves

Do you continually lose weight, then find it again? Here's a way to lose it effortlessly and keep it lost.

Picture yourself waking up in your bed at whatever time you usually awaken. Maybe you cast a sleepy eye at the clock and hunker back down under the covers for a few minutes. When you do decide to get up, push back the covers and swing your legs over the side of the bed. Something feels different.

Your body feels lighter. You lift your legs. Yup, definitely lighter there. You put your hand on your stomach. Yup, there too. You must be dreaming. You look around for an answer, and notice that the bed is littered with crumbs. They look like cookie crumbs, or cracker crumbs, or cake crumbs, but bigger.

Just then a brigade of elves marches onto your bed carrying brooms, shovels, and wicker baskets. You know that they're elves because on the front of each one's jerkin is embroidered the word *Elf*. They're whistling a jaunty tune, and as they pass by, you see the word *Fat* embroidered on the back of their jerkins.

Without so much as a howdy-do they set to work, sweeping the crumbs into a pile, then shoveling them into baskets. Wait just a calorie-pickin' minute—what's going on here? Tap one of the elves on his little shoulder and demand an explanation. The elf plucks his cap from his curly head, and bows to you. "Greetings and salutations," he says in a high voice. "We're the Fat Elves, at your service."

"What in the world of weight are you talking about?" you ask.

The little Fat Elf realizes that this is all new to you, and adopts a patient expression. He explains their activities to you as if talking to someone who's been hiding out on a remote Pacific island, thinking that World War II is still going on. "We harvest fat. As soon as you began thinking thin, we were alerted that you were ripe. Weight is dropping from you all through the day and—as in this case—all through the night. We collect your fat—wherever you are—and take it with us. You lose; we gain."

You take in this information, and digest it. "But what do *you* do with it?"

"We use it for compost—you should see our flowers and berry bushes—and feed it to our pets. If someone becomes way too thin, we give him some."

At first your mind boggles at the idea, but you quickly warm to it. "You mean that just because I've been thinking thin, I'm actually losing weight?"

With as much patience as he can muster, the little Fat Elf says, "That's the idea." Then laughs and slaps his little knee. "Get it? 'That's the *idea*,'" and laughs some more. You must look puzzled, because the elf explains. "It's the *idea* of being thin that makes your body lose weight. And we're here to make sure it stays lost." Then in a conspiratorial whisper, the elf says, "In case you didn't know, the Weight War is over."

"Well, thank you very much," you say to all the Fat Elves. And to yourself you think: well, well, well, this thinking thin is indeed a fine idea! To think that my body digests food efficiently—and it does—is a splendid idea. And to think that the food eaten turns to energy instead of fat—and it does—is a lovely idea.

Whistling a jaunty tune, you get dressed, noticing that your clothes fit just a bit looser. You have breakfast. The brigade of Fat Elves marches in and shovels up the fat you dropped, and as a bonus they get some of the crumbs from breakfast, too.

If you want to know how much you're losing, the elves can put their baskets of fat on a scale and weigh them. But they only like to do this once in a while, because if the amount lost is small, you might become discouraged and overeat, causing them to lose fat, and you to gain it.

To avoid this problem, some Fat Elves have a scale that simply reads Enough. They'd rather that you look at the big picture of you losing small amounts of weight on a regular basis over a period of time. Then you can measure your weight loss by how loose your clothes are, or the number of compliments you receive, or how good you feel about yourself and life.

Whatever you do during the day, wherever you go, the Fat Elves are there to collect the weight you lose. They sweep fat crumbs from the seat of your car, or the bus, or the subway. They're on the jogging path and at the office, the conference room, the lunch table, the gym, the dry cleaner's, the grocery store, the dinner table, on the television chair, and in bed.

They're everywhere, because you lose weight everywhere, every day and night. After every activity—no matter how passive or active—picture the brigade of Fat Elves marching in and shoveling your crumbs of lost fat into wicker baskets. Toss them a few extra crumbs from time to time, but once you've lost weight—don't try to find it!

Thinabration

Fat is out! Out of your mind. Out of your body. Out of your life.

Thin is in! In your mind. In your body. In your life. It's time to celebrate!

Where do you want to hold your Thinabration? Choose an environment that makes you feel good about yourself and about life. A place that brings a smile to your face. It could be as simple as your kitchen to show that you've triumphed over the lures of the refrigerator, or in a restaurant to flaunt your victory over overeating. How about aboard a cruise ship on the high seas, or high in the sky aboard a jumbo jet?

Host the party in an outdoor spot that you find especially beautiful and inspiring. If you can't think of a place you know, think of a place you'd like to know and create it in your mindscape. Feeling fanciful? Have your Thinabration on another planet in a far galaxy of your mind. Or on a cloud because you're so light. Or at the end of a rainbow because life is golden.

Whatever the party environment you choose, bring it to life in your mind. Picture or sense the details. Is the surface you're standing on hard or soft, rough or smooth? Notice the temperature of the air against your skin. Is it dry or moist? What aromas does the air carry? What sounds? Make the details as vivid and colorful as possible.

Now decorate your party place. Somewhere, draped across the refrigerator or flying from the cloud, there's a large banner proclaiming, CONGRATULATIONS: (YOUR NAME) IS HAPPILY THIN. What color is the banner? What color and shape are the letters? As you read the words on the banner your heart thumps with pleasure. Your mind glows with pride.

What other decorations do you want? Flowers? The tablecloth, plates, and napkins can display the words *Thin Is In* in a pleasant design. Are you going to use silverware or goldware? How about goblets?

Make out the guest list. Whom do you want to invite to your celebration party? Invite people who love you and who supported your desire to lose weight. They might be family members, friends, and coworkers. Invite anyone who helped you develop healthy eating habits and exercise routines. You might invite your doctor, or nutritionist, or physical trainer. Invite anyone and everyone who is truly glad to see you slim, fit, and healthy. See their names on the guest list.

What are you going to serve your guests? When you plan the menu, make it both healthy and fun. For instance, have both fruit and cake. After all, when you're thinking thin you can have your cake and eat it, too, because you're in control and will eat only a healthy amount.

You've picked the place for your party, selected the decorations, set the table, made a guest list, and planned the menu. Survey all that you've created. If there's anything you want to add, subtract, or change, do so.

When all is ready, see yourself at the place you've created for your celebration, and feel yourself there. What are you wearing? What design is it? Make it something flattering that shows off your new contours. What color is your celebration outfit? What material is it made of? Brush it with your hand and feel the texture. Excitement bubbles up inside you. Let the Thinabration begin!

The guests you've invited begin to arrive. You greet your first guest, and he or she gives you a warm smile and a huge hug, saying how great you look. Then he or she hands you a present. It might be a plant, a pet, or something wrapped up in a box. Each guest greets you warmly and brings you a gift. Receive your gifts with heartfelt thanks.

What kinds of festive clothes are your co-celebrators wearing? They might have on their best party clothes, or they might arrive in costumes from the past or the future. They could be festooned in ruffles, or satin, or glitter.

One guest arrives bringing a magician as his or her gift to you. The magician has a kind face, and his blue eyes brim with wisdom. How is he dressed? How tall is he? You aren't limited to one, or even three wishes, because this magician lets you know that he'll grant your wishes now and in the future. You're almost overwhelmed with possibilities. Your first wish is that the Thinabration is a merry experience for all. Your second wish is that each guest be granted a wish. And your third wish is to remain thin. What's your fourth wish?

By now all your guests have arrived, and your celebration party is well underway. The band strikes up one
of your favorite songs, and you dance with one of the
guests. You're light on your feet and dance with graceful
energy. Your guests join you on the dance floor. Everyone
is having a splendid time.

Having worked up an appetite dancing, everyone sits
down at the long banquet table to eat. The food servers
are animals: dogs, cats, goats, cows, elephants, bears,
lions, and giraffes. Maybe a hippopotamus. Each one
wears a bow-tie, or has an apron tied around its waist.

The serving animals circulate around the table bearing platters heaped with delicious-looking healthy food.
The guests help themselves to the food they want. You
help yourself to the food you want, too, taking only as
much as you know you can comfortably eat.

Next comes the champagne and sparkling cider. The
serving animals fill everyone's goblet with bubbly golden
liquid, and the guests begin, one by one, to toast you.
Each guest holds his or her goblet high, looks lovingly
into your eyes, and proposes a toast. They toast your thinness, your health, your courage, your intelligence, your
strength, your gentleness, and your spirit.

With love and sincerity the guests toast all the things
about you that they like and admire, and after each toast
there is a robust round of applause and cheering whistles.
Each word that you hear gladdens your heart beyond
measure. Knowing that your family and friends appreciate
who you are and what you've accomplished touches you
so that tears of joy gather and spill. You feel as if you

have feasted on love and are so nourished and full that food is but a remote and secondary consideration.

Holding your own goblet high, you toast your family and friends, thanking them for their help, love, and support. You tell them how great it feels to be thin. That being thin is fun and makes you happy. That you did it, and are doing it!

When you're finished speaking, everyone applauds and whistles. A troupe of clowns enters doing somersaults and cartwheels, and there's not a sad-faced one in the bunch. They take down the banner that proclaims, CON-GRATULATIONS: (YOUR NAME) IS HAPPILY THIN, and wave it exuberantly as they clown around the banquet table. Then the clowns, skipping and jumping, bring the banner over to you and drape it around you. You are happily thin for all to see. What a grand and glorious Thinabration!

Do this visualization as often as you want both to encourage yourself to lose weight, and to celebrate the weight you lose. The more you celebrate your success, the more success you'll have to celebrate.